The Secret Sex Lives of Older Women

Judy Higgs

Printed in Australia
Editing by Green Olive Press
Cover Design by Fiona Mearon
ISBN: 978-1-7644659-0-8

This book is dedicated to the women who trusted me with stories that they had long kept to themselves. This book exists because of your courage, your laughter, and for reminding all of us that intimacy and connection do not have an expiry date.

THE SECRET SEX LIVES OF OLDER WOMEN

Judy Higgs

I

Introduction

How it All Began

"The lady in the red top in the front row—what kind of book do you want to write?"

Not the kind of question a woman hopes to hear when she has arrived late, flustered, and planning to blend into the background like a potted plant. My friend and I had tiptoed into our first writing class only to discover that the back row—the sanctuary of the shy, the unsure, and the hungover—was full. The front row was all that remained. I smiled politely at Isobel, our writing-group coordinator, while silently checking the available exits.

"I was thinking about writing something on… grandparenting," I said, in the voice of someone hoping the fire alarm might go off and rescue her.

From behind me came a theatrical groan. "Dull, dull, dull."

I swivelled around to identify the heckler.

"Oh? And what would you suggest?" I asked.

He didn't hesitate. "Write about older women and their sex lives."

The room went still. Faces turned towards me, expectant, waiting.

Instead of laughing or fainting or reporting him to the UN, I heard myself say:

"Alright then. Challenge accepted."

And just like that, everything changed. One moment, I was a grandmother toying with the idea of a perfectly respectable book about bedtime routines and recipes for scones; the next, I had accepted a dare that plunged me headlong into sex, intimacy, and everything polite society prefers older women not to mention.

I realised I needed to talk to women my own age about their private lives. Tentatively at first—close friends over coffee, then friends of friends, neighbours, neighbours' sisters, and eventually anyone who stood still long enough. They, in turn, ushered me towards other women, and the circle widened.

Before long, I was being entrusted with written accounts from women aged sixty-two to ninety-one—stories that were startlingly honest, unapologetic, and often very funny. What struck me most was not just what they revealed, but their relief. Someone, at last, wanted the truth—not the stereotype.

My reading habits shifted accordingly. I searched bookshops and libraries for anything on ageing and intimacy. Once, when I queried an overdue book, the librarian began reading my borrowing history aloud. Halfway through, she faltered and lowered her voice, but by then the entire library knew exactly what I'd been reading. I didn't mind. I was far too engrossed to feel embarrassed.

Because this was no longer a mildly eccentric pastime. It was becoming a mission.

Along the way, I met extraordinary women—ordinary women, really, but with exceptional candour. They shared stories that were tender, raw, funny, and deeply human. In telling them, they felt seen and heard, and I began to understand just how invisible the world so often makes women over sixty.

For me, this journey has felt nothing short of a pilgrimage. It has shocked my children—and I suspect it will continue to do so. But the thought that delights me most is this: one day, I hope one of my grandchildren will announce at school, with pride, "My granny has written a sex book."

An Unspoken Adventure

We hear a great deal about sex, mostly about younger people under forty. Meanwhile, a vast and growing group is quietly excluded from the conversation. Older women, it seems, are expected to slip into a polite kind of invisibility.

There are nearly four hundred million women over the age of sixty five worldwide, a figure projected to almost triple by 2050. And yet their intimate lives remain largely unexamined. Is it because sex in later life is taboo? Or because it is assumed that older women simply lose interest? They do not. But their desire has become a secret—one rarely shared, even among friends.

This book exists to break that silence.

The Secret Sex Lives of Older Women asks an unfashionable question: why shouldn't Granny have a lover? Or a girlfriend? Or an appetite for pleasure that hasn't expired simply because she now qualifies for a senior's card?

The stories in this book are real. They belong to women who have lived full, complex lives—through marriage and divorce, widowhood and new love, illness, abstinence, affairs, and rediscovery. Some spent years without sex; others became more adventurous once long relationships ended. Many had affairs, some with married men. What unites them is not recklessness, but honesty—and a quietly radical acceptance of their own sexuality.

These women came of age during a period of extraordinary social change. They marched, protested the Vietnam War, danced to the Beatles, took the pill, wore miniskirts, burned bras, stayed out all night, and still turned up for work the next morning. Desire did not disappear with age; it evolved. And their stories prove that longing does not retire—it adapts.

I spoke with women aged sixty-five to ninety—or, as Maria Rosa proudly corrected me, eighty-nine and three-quarters. They spoke with warmth, wit, and astonishing candour. Secrets long buried surfaced with relief. Again and again, I heard the same response: At last, someone is talking about us—older women.

A few brave male friends also shared their experiences. After much consideration, I decided to include them. After all, if we are going to have sex with men, it helps to understand how they experience intimacy too.

Growing up in the 1950s and 1960s shaped how many women learned—or failed to learn—about sex. Pleasure was mysterious, often shameful, and rarely discussed. Women's desire barely rated a mention. That silence has consequences, many of which linger well into later life.

In the chapters that follow, I explore what has been hidden for too long: women's arousal and pleasure; men's emotional and physical experiences of intimacy; shifting libidos; long marriages that have gone stale; and the quiet question many women ask themselves—have I already had sex for the last time? I also examine love and intimacy in aged care, where desire persists even when privacy does not.

This is not a how-to manual promising better orgasms by page seventy-three. It is something more complex—and more honest. It is about need, connection, pleasure, and the right to desire without shame.

This book may challenge what you think you know about love, sex, and growing older. My hope is that it also offers permission: to speak openly, to support one another, to seek what we want— whether that is companionship, passion, or a better vibrator— without guilt or embarrassment.

Because sexuality does not end just because the calendar says it should.

II

What Do Older Women Really Want?

"Getting old is the second-biggest surprise of my life, but the first, by a mile, is our unceasing need for deep attachment and intimate love."—Roger Angell

"I'm eighty, and I've closed up shop down there." Jane Fonda stunned audienc.es when she said this in an interview for *The Guardian* about *The Book Club*. Shock, horror—an older woman talking about sex in a complete sentence. No coy euphemisms, no apologising. Just candour.

And perhaps she was right. For some women in their sixties and seventies, sex is no longer important. For others, later life marks the beginning of a new and unexpected adventure—sometimes the best sex of their lives.

Meet Sharon.

Like Jane Fonda, Sharon had firmly closed up shop. Then she met Stephen. A spark she assumed had long gone flickered back to life. Instead of collecting grandchildren from school and dispensing tea and cake, she found herself, gin and tonic in hand, stretched beside a pool while a retired doctor applied sunscreen to her back with unmistakable intent.

You may not recognise yourself in either story. Most women

sit somewhere in between.

How we feel about sex in our sixties and seventies is rarely how we felt in our twenties, thirties, or forties—particularly after menopause. For some, freedom from contraception, careers, and noisy teenagers creates space for a new era of intimacy, sometimes with a new partner. For others, sex feels like a closed chapter.

Have you shut up shop too?

Or do you sometimes think wistfully about the intimacy and closeness you once shared?

Chances are, you haven't spoken about it—not with your doctor, your partner, or even your closest friend. And yet why shouldn't it be discussed? Why shouldn't women share experiences and learn from one another?

After sixty, we enter a new stage of life. Pregnancy is no longer a concern. Our partners have changed too. The young Lochinvars who once roared up on motorbikes or Vespas, clad in black leather and full of promise, are now navigating footpaths on mobility scooters in their favourite slippers.

But does that mean we are done with sex? Apparently not.

One survey reports that 68 per cent of married men and thirty eight per cent of married women over seventy describe their sex lives as active and satisfying. Numbers aside, what mattered more to me were the stories.

There was Gwen, who met a recent widower. What began as companionship turned into love—to the astonishment of them both.

"I'm surprised by how much I enjoy being courted," she told me. "I believed what everyone says about older women—that we're past love and desire. It's simply not true."

Which raised a bigger question. Are women missing sex itself—or intimacy?

As I listened to these stories, a pattern emerged. Outwardly, lives had changed. Internally, women felt much the same as they always had. They talked freely about sex—or the absence of it— about their partners' difficulties, the mechanics, the frequency. But underneath it all, the longing was not just for sex.

It was for intimacy. For touch. For being valued.

Women, at heart, are not complicated. We want to be desired.

And that, frankly, is far more arousing than any unsolicited photograph of male anatomy could ever be.

Susan, whose sex life ended when her husband was diagnosed with prostate cancer, explained that it wasn't the loss of sex she grieved most—it was the loss of closeness. Touch faded. Connection waned. The physical expression of intimacy disappeared, and with it something vital.

I was reminded of this when I accompanied a close friend—eighty on her last birthday—to a surgical consultation for a hip replacement. As the appointment drew to a close, the surgeon asked if she had any questions.

I stared out the window, trying not to engage in this personal conversation.

After a discreet cough, she asked, "How soon after surgery can I resume sexual relations with my partner?"

To his credit, the surgeon smiled wryly.

"Whenever you're comfortable, Mrs Kendall—though perhaps wait until you're home."

Sex is not love, as Jay Shetty reminds us. But for many women, sex is one of the ways intimacy is sustained.

So why do some women shut up shop?

Familiarity and boredom featured often. Intimacy can become routine. Sex begins to feel like a chore rather than a pleasure. Pauline, for one, was delighted to be alone at last—liberated from disappointing sex and finally living for herself.

For others, a partner's erectile dysfunction marked a turning point. Sex became fraught. Some women still wanted intimacy but felt unable to raise the subject, fearing embarrassment or injury to fragile egos. And so, silence prevailed.

But why should that signal the end of intimacy?

Many women argued it shouldn't—and needn't. Sex, they said, does not have to involve a penis. While erections may matter deeply to men, women often experience desire differently. This raises an intriguing possibility: might there be a new model of sex in later life?

One not focused on performance or penetration. One centred on connection, pleasure, and erotic friendship.

If a penis misbehaves, that is not a woman's fault—nor her responsibility. Intimacy is not a mechanical exercise. It is about connection.

Even when sex ends—through illness, death, or choice—the need for touch and desire does not. Women still want to feel wanted. Even if we know we are no longer what we were in youth, we want to feel it anyway.

That is the secret of women's sexuality. And yet society no longer sees us. We become invisible—even to ourselves.

III

Still Sexy After All These Years

"I used to be the star of this show; now I've got a walk-on part."

If you believe everything you read, women become invisible shortly after menopause.

I certainly feel it. Standing at a family barbecue, scraping plates into the dishwasher while the conversation swirls around you, and wondering—what the fuck happened? I used to be the star of the show. Now I hover at the edges, playing minor roles in lives I once directed.

Perhaps we're meant to accept it. That's the circle of life, after all. But even when you understand it intellectually, it still hurts.

No wonder we feel a small thrill when someone actually notices us.

Gwen told me this when she described finding romance in her eighties. By then, she had almost given up, assuming she was nearing the final chapter of her life.

"It's not what we've always believed about older women," she said. "Octogenarians and romance don't exist in the media—not in magazines, newspapers, or online."

After Gwen was widowed at seventy-eight, she experienced several romances. None resembled the great love she shared with her husband, but that didn't diminish their value. She enjoys intimacy differently now. Sharing her bed with another warm body, she told me, is "every bit as wonderful."

Gwen is living proof that desire does not evaporate with age—it changes form.

Many women describe becoming invisible around the time they become grandmothers. But it's not just grandmothers; it's older women in general. And, interestingly, men told me they experience it too.

An eminent surgeon I know—an international prize-winner, a leader in his field—confided that after sixty, he felt increasingly unheard. Junior doctors' eyes glazed over as he spoke. Some were blunt enough to say, "We don't think that's relevant anymore." Yesterday's man. Time to move on.

Yet time and again, his experience triumphed. He diagnosed what others missed because he listened. His expertise hadn't vanished—it simply wasn't valued.

No one likes their identity threatened. Men, in particular, often define themselves by their work. When retirement strips away status and authority, it can be deeply destabilising. Alice observed that men born after 1945—department heads, CEOs, surgeons, lawyers—often struggle profoundly once their titles disappear.

And where are the dashing heroes of our youth now?

The actors who once made our hearts race now reappear on our TV screens selling incontinence pads, funeral plans, and devices to keep muscles active. It must sting—once the romantic leads whose photographs adorned bedroom walls are now ambassadors for old age.

Age humbles everyone. And yet shame seems to attach itself particularly to women.

"The trouble with getting older isn't the creaky knees," someone once said. "It's your own children acting like the food police." They peer into your fridge, tutting at yoghurt tubs as though they're radioactive. Never mind that many of us grew up eating tinned food stored since the war—and survived. Somehow, our entire generation walks around feeling vaguely guilty, as though even our groceries are moral failings.

And if we feel ashamed about yoghurt, what hope is there for sexuality?

Meet Hazel.

A widow after a long and happy marriage, Hazel sat down

at our local café and announced she had a problem. I assumed it involved grandchildren misbehaving on her white sofa, as usual, with chocolate biscuits. Instead, she told me she was lonely.

She had met a widower at church. They drank coffee together. She missed being hugged. She missed companionship. She wasn't looking for marriage, but she had started spending the night at his place. And her children were appalled.

They couldn't bear the thought of their mother dating anyone but their father. Hazel felt ashamed—not because she'd done anything wrong, but because society does not want to imagine older women as sexual beings.

Older women are invisible.

We are told—subtly and relentlessly—that we lose social and sexual currency as we age. That our value lies in childcare and casseroles. Some writers challenge this. Kathy Lette skewers ageing with humour; Emma Thompson's recent film, *Good Luck to You Leo Grande* (2022), explored an older woman's sexual awakening. But generally, sex belongs to the young and beautiful.

Older women rarely appear in advice columns or erotic fiction. We are absent even from conversations about desire. Is it any wonder we doubt our appeal?

And yet, when I met Maria Rosa, she told me something extraordinary.

At ninety, after a long and fulfilling sex life, this was the first time she had ever spoken about it to anyone. As we talked, her life unfolded—children, widowhood, grief, and even a love affair. Curious by nature, she had spent decades reading about women's sexuality.

"I feel more enlightened now than ever," she said. "I even know about things I never imagined—masturbation, vibrators."

When I first searched for books about women my age, I expected wisdom. What I found was wrinkle cream. Shelf after shelf offered ways to look younger, thinner, fresher. Sex—if mentioned at all—was whispered, apologised for, or hidden.

Meanwhile, youth itself has become an exhausting performance. Women in their twenties and thirties go to extraordinary lengths just to appear desirable.

Liz Jones, the award-winning journalist for the *Daily Mail*, has written candidly about the hours and expense poured into preparing for dates—hair removal, colouring, manicures, pedicures—until she resembles, she says, a pre-pubescent girl.

That is the formula: don't look old. But here is the truth.

Older women are still sexual beings. Not all of us—but many more than society acknowledges. And because we grew up with different myths, taboos, and silences to those of our daughters or our mothers, our experience of intimacy is uniquely complex.

Which brings us to the real question.

If desire doesn't disappear, why are we so determined to pretend it does?

IV

Growing up in the Fifties and Sixties

> "Most elderly participants in surveys on sexual behaviour developed their views during the early part of the twentieth century and could be expected to have different views from those born later."—Susan Deacon

Who else is in bed with you?

Quite a few things, as it turns out. Institutions. Religion. Schools. Social class. Social norms. And—perhaps most influential of all—our parents.

What we learned about sex, and just as importantly, what we didn't learn, continues to shape how we think about intimacy today. For those of us born in the post-war baby boom, our attitudes were forged at a peculiar crossroads: raised by parents formed by war and deprivation, yet coming of age during one of the most radical cultural shifts in modern history.

We were told one thing. The world then showed us another.

The Baby Boomer generation is often described as revolutionary, and in many ways that is true. We challenged politics, music, fashion, and authority. We believed we were breaking free from constraints that had shaped our parents' lives.

And yet there remains one stubborn taboo: the idea that

older adults might still want, enjoy, or seek sex.

Sex among older people is still treated as faintly ridiculous, faintly disgusting, or best whispered about behind closed doors. Open a newspaper or watch television and sex in later life is usually played for laughs—or shame. The suggestion that older adults might still desire intimacy often provokes embarrassment or outright revulsion.

We've lived through decades of change. So why does the idea of boomers continuing to explore love and intimacy seem so foreign? Maybe it's time we reframe the narrative. Our generation has always pushed boundaries, and maybe, just maybe, it's time we challenge this outdated perception as well.

Do they think we simply… stop? Newsflash: we may be older, but we are not dead.

Which makes it worth asking: how did we end up here?

Sex Education for the Beatles Generation

When we were growing up, sex education barely existed. There was no internet, no pornography at the click of a button, no dating apps, no casual talk of pleasure. There was no pill, no legal abortion, and homosexuality was not an option—it was a crime or a diagnosis.

In the UK, sex education was tentatively introduced into schools in the 1950s, to the horror of some parents who wrote furious letters to headmasters. Perhaps they felt children should learn about sex the traditional way—behind bike sheds, through whispers and misinformation.

In fairness, sex simply wasn't discussed in polite society. Books, plays, and films ended firmly at the bedroom door.

At my school, we officially learned about sex in our first year of secondary education. There was a hum of excitement. We quizzed the year above us for information because this was going to be the highlight of the academic year.

It wasn't called sex education. It was called reproductive biology in humans.

The emphasis was entirely on procreation—and it scared us girls shitless.

The task of sex education naturally fell to the biology teacher. We all adored Miss Violet Short, though she could be formidable. She wanted every one of us to go to Cambridge, where she had studied, and somehow she made it seem possible.

Miss Short was ahead of her time. She wore trousers and tailored jackets, had short hair, and had served in the Land Army during the war. She made no secret of her view that men were not essential. Air-raid wardens, she said, were particularly useless— too fond of themselves and no help at all during blackouts.

She was immensely popular with the girls. Probably one of the most respected teachers in the whole school.

When she wasn't supervising crayfish dissections, she taught us about sexual reproduction. In a classroom full of almost certainly virginal schoolgirls, she explained intercourse as the moment when the penis filled with blood, became a rigid rod, broke through the hymen, and penetrated the vagina. All the while, tapping the penis on a brightly coloured anatomy poster with her blackboard pointer.

We were fascinated... and terrified.

The girl beside me fled the room. We later learned she had fainted in the corridor and was revived by the sports mistress with hot, sweet tea.

At lunchtime, we sat in the canteen and debated whether marriage was worth it. After all, one wasn't supposed to have sex unless married. Eventually, we compromised: we'd wait and see—and perhaps wear pyjamas to bed on our wedding nights, as if that might help. We were eager for information and plied each girl who said they had had sex for the details. None were very forthcoming, and we learned nothing of any use. It was all rather vague and, as likely as not, made up. Probably, the one girl who could have told us quite a bit had left suddenly at the beginning of the term.

Teenage Boys and The Library

Boys, of course, were left largely to their own devices.

Before the internet, sex for teenage boys was a mystery—but boys determined to understand sex always find a way. My cousin Adrian recalls cycling home from school in the 1960s when an older boy asked him, "Have you had a wank yet?"

Too embarrassed to ask what a wank was, Adrian cycled straight to his local library. In the reference section, he pulled down *Encyclopaedia Britannica*, he found the WXYZ volume, and read: "Wank: a slang term for masturbation."

No wiser, because he didn't know what masturbation was, he carefully replaced the WXYZ volume and searched under "M". Eventually, he found the entry labelled 'masturbation'.

Thus began his self-directed sexual education.

Patricia Campbell, author of *Sex Education Books for Young Adults, 1892-1979*, said, "Although parents and schools should be the basic providers of sound sex education, they seldom are. This leaves the library as the only source of sex education for young people."

Even today, education often misses the mark. When I asked two teenage members of my own family about sex education, they remembered an early anatomy lesson they barely understood— and soon forgot. What stayed with them was a later session led by a GP who spoke less about body parts and more about relationships.

They felt year eleven would have been the right time for meaningful discussion. Unfortunately, final school exams intervened, and that was the end of their sex education.

The boys added that there was a slight flurry of talking about sex during the #MeToo movement, but discussions remained basic. While the headmaster thought this was essential to their education, probably under media pressure, the boys felt that asking for consent came naturally. They admitted that they had viewed porn at some time, but they never discussed this with their parents, so nobody told them that porn wasn't much like the relationships they would have with partners.

If not parents or grandparents, who should be having these conversations?

Sex, Social Class, and Lady Chatterley

When we were young, so much was forbidden—especially anything indecent. The book that electrified teenage curiosity was *Lady Chatterley's Lover*.

It wasn't just the sex. It was sex across class boundaries. Pregnancy without marriage. Words like fuck and cunt. And perhaps most shocking of all: an explicit description of female pleasure.

When Penguin republished the novel in 1960 after its obscenity trial, Baby Boomers were in their teens, hormonal and ravenous for information. The book sold millions.

It told a tender love story alongside graphic sex—a revelation for a generation raised on silence. That was a lot for our generation, the Baby Boomers, to unravel.

No wonder we feel guilty about sex; look what we had to go through. And then there was religion.

V

God, Sex, and What Will the Neighbours Say?

> "Religion is regarded by the common people as true, by the wise as false, and by rulers as useful."—Seneca, 4BC-AD 65

If you want to understand why so many older women struggle to speak openly about sex, don't start in the bedroom. Start in childhood.

Because, in addition to being influenced by sex education in school, we were also taught about sex through the veil of religion. Because for those of us who grew up in Britain in the 1950s and 1960s, church wasn't just something you did on Sunday. It was a lens through which you viewed the world—and a fog through which you viewed sex. School taught us biology. Religion taught us shame. Society added a final warning: and don't you dare let the neighbours find out. No wonder it still clings to us.

Smells and Bells: Being Catholic in the Sixties

When I was sixteen and living in Canada, my boyfriend David's parents invited me to dinner. It was freezing outside, the kind of cold that requires a small mountain of coats, scarves, and boots—items you peel off at the door like armour, because Canadians keep their heating turned up to tropical.

David's mother ushered me into her bedroom to leave my winter paraphernalia. I noticed immediately there was no shared marital bed—just two single beds, neatly made.

I found out why later.

Their house was nothing like my post-war brick box of a home. This place was bohemian: brass rubbings from Chartres Cathedral nestled among Native American artwork. The family was devoutly Catholic, intelligent, and utterly fascinating. David's brother—training for the priesthood—joined us for dinner, and the conversation drifted, as it often did in Catholic circles, towards sex while pretending not to.

That night, it was contraception.

At the time, the only "approved" method for Catholics was the rhythm method: tracking cycles, predicting ovulation, and abstaining when pregnancy was most likely. The theory was moral; the reality was a tense calendar and a great deal of anxiety.

Couples like David's parents slept in separate beds during the "fertile window"—not for the woman's comfort, but to prevent the husband being "tempted."

David's parents were doctors, so they took a keen interest

in this debate. The conversation crept deep into the night. They discussed Dr John Rock, a devout Catholic doctor they both knew and who taught at Harvard Medical School. He would become one of the leading clinical researchers responsible for developing the pill. While a firm Catholic, Dr Rock strongly supported using the contraceptive pill for Catholic women. Unfortunately, not everyone felt this way, particularly the Pope.

It was, as so much of it was, built around men's needs and men's weakness—never women's desire.

Information was scarce. Questions felt dangerous. Maria Rosa, living in Australia at the time, confirmed this, "Contraception before—and even after marriage—was complex. It was so hard to get information about how to use it. We would never have asked even our doctor."

"As Catholics, we were taught intimacy before marriage was a mortal sin," she told me. "So the pill—though newly introduced—was beyond our reach. The rhythm method was the only option, which meant abstaining when you were ovulating… except I didn't have a regular cycle, so I never actually knew when that was."

Mark, one of my male contributors, was sceptical when asked whether the rhythm method works.

"Well," he said, "we went on to have three more children."

Sometimes a punchline carries more truth than a sermon.

How Religion Makes Women Second-Class Citizens

Catholicism was not the only faith tradition in which women's lives were narrowed by rules, reproduction, and the expectation of obedience. Rachel's story—told through the lens of Orthodox Judaism—made that painfully clear.

Rachel is deeply engaged with her religion. After years in Australia, much of it as a single mother, she reflected on how profoundly religion had shaped her married life—especially sexually. Her second husband was raised in a world of strict observance, where rules governed everything from food to prayer to the body.

And in his daily morning prayers, wrapped in his tallit and facing away from ordinary life, he would give fervent thanks to God "for not making him a woman."

Few sentences provoke discomfort like that one.

Even if a scholar argues it's an ancient text, mistranslated, misunderstood—its impact is not subtle. Young boys hear it.

Boys repeat it. Men absorb it. And women live inside its shadow.

Rachel did. "Throughout the years," she told me, "I struggled to maintain my sense of self-worth, independence, happiness, and fulfilment—especially sexual. I learned to walk in his shadow. I was there to ensure his happiness, his fulfilment, his desire. I don't remember him being concerned enough to explore mine."

Modesty—tzniut—was the foundation of her world. Modesty meant dress, behaviour, reserve. A modest woman, she explained, makes an ideal mate. Even hair became private property. Married women covered theirs with scarves or wigs—sheitels—, so the world could not "see" what belonged to the husband.

Of course, modern life has its own delicious contradictions: some of the wigs are so stylish they look better than natural hair. Ancient rules, updated for contemporary vanity—still the same message underneath: your body is not quite your own.

Sex, Society, and Submission

Religion was only part of it. Society policed women's sexuality just as efficiently.

For our generation—and more truthfully, for our mothers— the guiding question was always the same:

What will the neighbours say?

Society tells us what to do. After the Second World War, the messages were blunt and consistent. From churches, parents, teachers, advertisements, books: don't do it before marriage. A woman who had sex outside marriage was "ruined." Her virginity was her "most valuable asset." Men might be excused. Women were punished.

And punishment was swift if it became visible.

If a woman became pregnant, she was often ostracised by her community because people at the time were acutely aware of what the neighbours would think. So, the poor pregnant girl, like the girl from my class at school, was shuffled off to distant relatives until the baby was born or to a mother-and-baby home run by a religious organisation. Alternatively, the parents arranged for a hasty shotgun wedding.

Society might tolerate promiscuity as a rumour, but not as a bump under a cardigan.

Pamela was one such "speedy bride."

"After my first experience of intercourse, I was pregnant," she said. "In the 1960s, we had to get married."

They married for society, not for love, and the marriage didn't last. Pamela became a single mother—punished twice: first for sex, then for the consequences.

And even now, in some parts of the world, the obsession with "purity" persists. Some women feel pressured to undergo surgery to "restore" the hymen—an attempt to satisfy cultural demands that are medically ignorant and psychologically brutal. A hymen is not proof of virginity. It can tear from sport, tampons, or ordinary life. Ignorance is dangerous—and shame is its weapon of choice.

The Neighbours and the Wedding Night

Sally and Richard were my next-door neighbours. Born just after the war, educated in single-sex schools, they belonged to that familiar world where sex existed everywhere and was discussed nowhere.

Unlike both their parents, who were born just after World War I, they did at least have some sex education at school and at home. Sally learned about boys' anatomy by changing her baby brother's nappy. Richard's education was no better. His father was killed in the war. His mother was too embarrassed to speak to her son about such matters. So, Richard's sex education came from vastly exaggerated stories of his friend's experiences in Welsh caravans during the school holidays.

Whilst Richard was keen to have sex before they got married, Sally was not so keen. She saw the shame that her cousin Ann and her best friend at school, Tess, experienced when their foray into premarital sex resulted in pregnancy. Society saw to it that these young women's potentially exciting young lives were cut short by the trauma of a forced adoption for Ann and an abortion for Tess. Sally was determined that this was not going to happen to her, and she decided that she wasn't going to have sex with Richard until she was married. It wasn't unusual for women during this time to remain virgins until their wedding night. Not that our grandchildren would believe that.

So they arrived at their wedding night innocent, anxious, and utterly unprepared. They didn't know the language of bodies. They'd never heard the word clitoris. Films still showed married couples sleeping in separate beds. The pill existed, but access was tightly controlled, and Sally had to persuade her GP she was "about to be married" to obtain it.

She left it a bit late to go to the doctor for her medication, so she and Richard had to use condoms, a present kindly left in their honeymoon room by Richard's best man. The best man had chosen some novelty condoms, different colours and apparently, they laughed so much trying to get the hang of them that they didn't manage to have sex that night.

It's a funny story—until you realise how much fear and ignorance it contains.

This notion of abstinence before marriage still exists in many parts of the world. For example, in 2022, the Indonesian parliament unanimously approved new laws that criminalise sex outside marriage. Eventually, the new laws may also apply to non-Indonesians living in the country for work, and perhaps even to tourists who holiday in Bali each year.

Neighbours Didn't Like Homosexuality Either.

And if society had rules for heterosexual women, it had harsher ones for anyone outside that script.

Long before legal reforms arrived, many gay people married under pressure: the nuclear family was the ideal, respectability was safety, and secrecy was survival. Women married men who could not desire them and so blamed themselves. They felt undesirable, defective, at fault.

Abigail speculated that, although she didn't know it then, all the signs were there that her husband was gay. She told me that if he had been honest from the start of the relationship, she might have handled it better. She was unaware of his secret sexuality, and she often felt she wasn't attractive enough for him to want to have sex with her. She had an affair almost to prove to herself that she was sexually attractive. "Forty years later, on reflection, I suspect that he may have been bisexual or gay, but such was my ignorance. I didn't have a clue what that meant. Growing up, I never knew about such things."

Rachel knew her husband was gay, but they were Orthodox Jews, and the religion disapproved of homosexuality, so they kept it a secret. She said, 'The 1980s also saw a significant shift towards the emergence of a global gay culture. "The marriage lasted a difficult eighteen years. Shrouded in the secrecy of my husband's struggle with his own hidden sexuality and dalliances."

When her husband later died of AIDS, she even found herself blamed—because in a culture built on shame, someone must always be at fault, and it is usually the woman.

For lesbians, the absence was total: no role models, no

language, no representation.

Society was slow to accept gay culture. There were no lesbian or butch role models on television or film, says award-winning poet Joelle Taylor and growing up as a lesbian had its difficulties. The available magazines, like *Jackie* and *Just Seventeen*, didn't talk about lesbians. The magazines told girls how to get a boyfriend—never a girlfriend. Some women only felt able to name their truth decades later, once society loosened its grip and legal change made a private life less dangerous.

We have moved on. Not far enough, perhaps—but enough that more women can now choose who they love, without living a double life.

Which brings us to the next question.

If we were trained from childhood to feel shame—about sex, about desire, about our own bodies—what do we actually know about how our bodies work? And if no one ever told us, how do we begin—now—to learn?

VI

Secret Women's Business

> "Women are responsible for their sexuality now. A woman's pleasure is not dependent upon the presence of a penis in the vagina; neither is a man's."— Germaine Greer

It is a truth universally acknowledged that a heterosexual woman in possession of a vagina must be in want of a penis.

Not Jane Austen's exact words, obviously — though she would have understood the economics behind the idea. In her world, a woman's survival often depended on attracting a man. Love was lovely, but financial security was the real romance.

Two hundred years on, we like to think we've moved beyond that. And we have—mostly. Yet when it comes to sex, the old script still lingers, men's pleasure at centre stage; women's pleasure as a supporting role. Sometimes it's ignored. Sometimes it's considered "nice if it happens." Sometimes it's treated as a bonus feature.

And that is where this chapter begins.

Because we older women are not making babies anymore. Sex, for many of us now, is not about reproduction. It is about pleasure, connection, and the right to enjoy our own bodies without apology.

Which raises an awkward question. If women's pleasure is

so central to women's sexuality, why were so many of us never told the basic facts?

The Beginning of the Pleasure Revolution

Sharon saw her marriage from a different perspective when she became a mature-age student at university. She describes how it affected the breakdown of her marriage. 'I began to see that society prioritised the male point of view—and that applied to my marriage.'

For centuries, sex research—like sex itself—was framed around function: procreation, erections, penetration, "performance." Women were present, of course, but mostly as the necessary environment for male activity.

Women's pleasure was not required to keep the species going, so it was conveniently treated as irrelevant.

But recently, researchers have begun to be less interested in the procreative mechanisms of sex and to turn their attention to the desire for sex. Why does it occur, and who gets turned on more quickly, and who loses interest sooner? While slow, the results are spectacular.

Sex, desire, and lust between people and particularly how it affects women, is the new focus of research. We never knew that sex could be fun.

No wonder so many of our mothers and grandmothers experienced sex as something endured rather than enjoyed. My grandmother, who gave birth to ten children, never struck me as someone who thought sex was "fun." It was more likely a duty, a risk, a dread—with an inevitable outcome.

Education failed us. Religion scolded us. And many of us stumbled into adulthood with no clear sense that pleasure was even on the menu. Maria Rosa still sounds indignant about the wasted years.

"We didn't understand lovemaking," she told me. "We didn't even know women had orgasms. In my generation—I'm eighty-nine—nobody talked about any of this."

And yet the world has shifted. Slowly. Unevenly. But unmistakably.

Books, films, whispered conversations with friends—they've all helped us wise up. And for that, we can thank two remarkable women. Professor Helen O'Connell, an Australian urologist, was the first to properly map the clitoris—the true epicentre of female pleasure. And Canadian psychologist Professor Meredith Chivers set out to chart the terrain of desire itself. Together, they lit the fuse on a revolution that is still smouldering.

And as it turns out, women's sexuality is nothing like we were taught to believe.

Arousal Isn't Desire—and That Changes Everything

One of the most liberating ideas in modern sex research is also the simplest: Arousal is not the same as desire.

We tend to lump them together, as if they're one thing. But they aren't. They sit on different branches of the tree.

Arousal can happen in the body without meaning. It doesn't mean that they are thinking… I want sex.

Desire, on the other hand, is personal. Contextual. Emotional. Sometimes inconvenient. Sometimes wildly absent at the worst possible moment and sometimes with the most inappropriate people.

This distinction matters because it helps explain something many women have experienced and felt ashamed about: the body responding when the mind is not remotely interested—or the mind being curious while the body is uncooperative.

It also explains why women's desire often has less to do with "visual stimulus" and more to do with mood, safety, connection, and whether anyone has left wet towels on the bed.

As Esther Perel has pointed out, women's interest can flare in the right conditions—or vanish without a trace. Men's arousal is often described as more straightforward, frequently tied to erections and performance. Women's desire, by contrast, is frequently a symphony: body, mind, mood, history, and circumstance all playing at once.

Which means treating women's sexuality like a plumbing problem is not only inaccurate—it's insulting.

"Female Sexual Dysfunction" and the Problem with Labels

If a woman's interest in sex fades, the world has a name for her. Frigid. Broken. Dysfunctional.

The worst insult you can give a woman is to suggest that she is frigid, that something is wrong with her for not wanting sex on demand. And because society loves a diagnosis—especially one that can be treated—women's shifting desire has increasingly been framed as a medical problem.

If women go off the idea of having sex with their partners, it is diagnosed as sexual dysfunction. Dr Edwar Laumann estimated that forty three percent of women have female sexual dysfunction. Yet, according to another health professional, it doesn't technically exist.

Clinical psychologist and renowned sexologist Lenore Tiefer contends that "there can be no treatments because there is no actual condition." She has long challenged the medical community's approach to diagnosing and treating sexual difficulties in women, arguing that many so-called sexual disorders are socially constructed rather than genuine medical conditions. She points out that inventing diseases to sell treatments has a long history. What makes "female sexual dysfunction" (FSD) different is how blatant it is. Rather than growing out of women's own experiences, it was shaped and pushed by corporate interests, turning natural changes in women's desire into something labelled as broken.

And so FSD was born. But many women's so-called "sexual dysfunction" isn't a disorder at all.

If it does not exist, why do we need treatment?

Well, it doesn't exist. It's a fraud. The British Medical Journal in described FSD in an editorial as the clearest example yet of the corporate-sponsored creation of a disease. There is no end to these invented diseases. I recently saw a reference for hypoactive sexual desire disorder—look that one up. Someone or something is creating a market for drugs for a disease that doesn't exist.

Enter Big Pharma.

If there were a pill to increase libido, would you take it?

Some women might. Some men would prefer their partners did. And of course, research continues. Testosterone has been trialled. Some studies suggest it may improve desire and pleasure for some women — and like all drugs, it comes with trade-offs and side effects.

Some doctors offer testosterone to raise libido in women and men. Naturally, there are advantages and disadvantages to everything, particularly a drug. In Melbourne, a study assessed the potential benefits and risks of testosterone treatment compared with a placebo. The results showed that testosterone might increase sexual function, sexual desire, sexual pleasure, arousal, orgasm and self-image. But before we all rush off to get some testosterone, it also leads to significant weight gain, excess body hair, and acne. No, a pubescent male teenager is not what we want to be. The oral testosterone also led to a significant increase in levels of LDL (the wrong type of cholesterol), which then gets us thinking about the risk of heart disease and stroke, because women's desire isn't a physical problem.

But there is a more radical possibility: Maybe women don't need fixing. Maybe the script does.

We Know More About the Moon Than the Clitoris

Let's talk about the clitoris.

Or rather, let's talk about how we didn't... talk about it, that is. Who knew about the clitoris? I survived four years of nurse training, including anatomy and physiology lectures, and the word never came up once.

Many women I spoke to admitted they couldn't confidently identify the clitoris on a diagram. One of the contributors, who was a doctor, could. The rest were a bit vague.

And these are educated women. Competent women. Women who have run households, raised children, built careers, managed crises, and survived loss.

How is it possible we can organise a family Christmas for sixteen people and still not be entirely sure how our own bodies work?

Part of the answer is astonishing: for decades, the clitoris was either minimised, misrepresented, or left out entirely from anatomy textbooks. When Professor Helen O'Connell mapped the full structure properly—showing it was far larger and more complex than the tiny "button" most of us were taught to imagine—the shock wasn't that she discovered it. The shock was that modern medicine had ignored it.

She has even said it wasn't properly represented in the textbooks when she was a medical student. No wonder women grew up believing their pleasure was mysterious, optional, or non-existent. As my friend Sharon confessed, she hadn't the faintest idea what it was actually for.

"I didn't know what an orgasm was until it unexpectedly happened to me."

It has been that way for years. The clitoris has long been shrouded in mystery, almost like an iceberg, because most of its largest and most significant parts are hidden from view. Dr

O'Connell's detailed drawings revealed that the internal clitoral body, divided into two parts, can be as long as nine centimetres. These parts wrap around the vagina and can fill with blood, much like the penis. Interestingly, she also clarified that the so-called G-spot is simply the closest part of the vaginal wall—it isn't a distinct anatomical feature. Whether you believe in it or not is up to you, but she is not convinced.

And here is the blunt truth that sets many women free the moment they hear it:

Most women do not orgasm from penetrative sex alone. Despite all the myths, few women can achieve orgasm without clitoral stimulation. Research tells us that around 80 percent of women do not orgasm from penetrative sex alone. Women receive pleasure primarily through the clitoris, the organ devoted solely to pleasure.

And yet generations of women assumed they were 'odd,' "difficult," or "wrong" because penetration didn't reliably deliver the fireworks. They kept quiet because sex wasn't discussed—not even with friends.

Silence breeds shame. And shame is a marvellous way to keep women compliant.

Faking It: The Great Female Courtesy

If you want proof that women have been managing men's feelings for decades, look no further than the fake orgasm.

The film *When Harry Met Sally* (1989) captured it perfectly. Harry, played by Billy Crystal, says that he doesn't believe any of the women he had slept with had ever faked an orgasm. Sally proved otherwise—loudly, theatrically, and in a crowded restaurant. The scene is hilarious, memorable, and enduring because women recognised the truth instantly.

The quote "I'll have what she's having" is ranked thirty third on the American Film Institute's list of the one hundred greatest movie quotes of all time. This line is delivered by Estelle Reiner, who incidentally was the mother of the film's director.

Women enjoyed the joke because they realised they were not the only ones faking orgasm. It was a "woman thing" and unbelievably empowering. Men who watched the film didn't get the joke. Women laughed because they realised they weren't alone.

Men often didn't get the joke—because most men, deep down, assume a woman wouldn't possibly need to fake with them.

So why do women fake it?

To protect a partner's pride.

To end sex quickly.

Because it feels easier than explaining.

Because "nice girls" don't articulate what they want.

Because they've never been told they're allowed to feel pleasure.

Others said they faked it so that sex would be over quickly, and they could get down to things that really needed to be done, like feeding babies, answering emails and knitting woolly jackets for distressed penguins.

Vanessa Feltz, aged sixty one, a journalist in the UK who writes about her life, bluntly says, 'It is the polite thing to do if you are not feeling it and the man has been beavering away.'

Polite. That word alone tells you everything.

But here is the turning point. This is no longer about being polite.

It is about older women understanding their bodies, naming their pleasure, and claiming the right to intimacy that serves them too. Pleasure that doesn't rely on performance. Pleasure that doesn't require penetration. Pleasure that doesn't centre a penis as the main event.

Women's pleasure is not a footnote.

And if we want to stop faking orgasms and start enjoying sex more fully, men need to understand this too, not as a criticism, but as liberation.

Which brings us neatly to the next chapter. Because if we are going to speak honestly about women's sexuality, we also need to understand men's—particularly in later life, when bodies change, confidence wobbles, and intimacy needs a new map.

That is where we go next.

VII
Secret Men's Business

"The man's role is to perform for the woman by bringing her to orgasm; when he loses confidence in his ability to do this, he no longer wants to have sex."—Barry McCarthy

Like many women, I have made mistakes trying to understand men—particularly their relationship with their penises.

Women talk about breasts, of course, but we can go days, months, even years without mentioning them. Men, on the other hand, seem unable to stop talking about penises, joking about them. Worrying about them and measuring them—metaphorically and otherwise. From locker rooms to late-night thoughts, a penis carries more psychological weight than most would admit.

For many men, the penis is not just an organ. It is identity. Proof. Power. Vulnerability. Success and failure rolled into one fragile package. And when it falters, so can everything else.

Erections: a problem and a joy

Puberty is a joyous discovery. In the TV series *Sex Education (2019)*, one episode revolves around the problems of erections occurring at all the wrong times for the show's star, teenager Otis.

Men are obsessed with size and function, and anything to do with the penis is an inside joke shared by men. Men and their erections are always a good topic of conversation. As Roger Moore, aka James Bond, always said to his leading ladies at the beginning of a movie: "I have to apologise to you now for what might happen in the close-up scenes; if I get an erection, I apologise, and if I don't, I also apologise."

Erections: Public, Private, and Fraught

Sex is never entirely private for men. Their success or failure is visible.

That visibility breeds anxiety. Once sex moves beyond adolescent experimentation, men carry an enormous burden: Will it work? Will it stay up? Will I fail? One faltering episode can lodge in the mind like a curse.

When Sex Equals Survival

Former Wimbledon tennis star John Lloyd, who was once married to one of the most famous tennis superstars of all time, Chris Evert, was talking to the surgeon who was about to operate on him for prostate cancer. When advised of the possible consequences of the surgery, he replied that he would rather die than survive without a sex life.

That level of terror raises a question many women quietly ask "Do all men feel this way?"

Not quite. Neurosurgeon and bestselling author Dr Henry Marsh offers a very different response. Diagnosed with terminal prostate cancer, he reflected that he did not miss his libido or erections at all—and in many ways felt relieved to be free of them. Sex, he wrote, had brought him misery in youth and contributed to the breakdown of his first marriage.

When undergoing androgen deprivation therapy, he joked to a nurse that the world might be a better place if all men were on it.

Yet reading his account, I couldn't help wondering about the silence around his partner. What did she lose? Or gain? Men's reflections on sex often centre on themselves—which is understandable—but intimacy is never a solo act.

The Long Decline (and the Great Myth)

The first generation of rock stars—born between 1940 and

1955—would have us believe that sexual prowess improves with age. It doesn't.

Biologically speaking, men peak early. Testosterone declines slowly but steadily from adolescence onward. Desire may persist, sometimes stubbornly, but performance becomes increasingly unreliable. And because men's arousal is visible, public, and measurable, failure is humiliating.

When the penis doesn't perform, many men don't simply lose sex—they lose confidence, identity, and desire itself.

Would Men be Reassured to Know that Most Women Care Far Less about Erections than Men Imagine?

Sharon, who at seventy-four began a relationship with a doctor her own age, put it plainly:

"His erectile dysfunction didn't bother me at all. It was the best sex I'd ever had. Sex doesn't have to revolve around erections or orgasms." What worried her more was how he felt about it.

Desire Is Not the Same as Function

Esther Perel has written extensively about this: when a man cannot achieve an erection, it strikes at his sense of self. She comments on the fragility of men's identities, explaining how difficult it is to develop them and how easy it is to lose them. Masculinity, for many men, has been carefully constructed—and is easily shattered.

The crucial distinction is this: A man may still want sex. He may still desire closeness.

But fear of failure stops him from trying.

The desire for sex for men is not the same as the function. In other words, it's possible to fix a man's ability to have sex physically, but his desire for sex is different. That desire can remain constant—even as he is ogling his carers in the nursing home, perhaps even when he has forgotten why. But being able to have sex is what gives him anxiety. For some men, the worry is not about wanting sex anymore but about whether they can.

Sometimes the desire remains long after the ability has faded—the body betraying the mind. Sometimes testosterone declines, and desire wanes too. And sometimes life intervenes with depression, anxiety, money worries, illness, and grief.

Because men, like women, are complex.

Is Your Partner 'the One In Four' with Low Testosterone?

Sometimes, the desire disappears. Testosterone is the petrol that fires the engine, and it was always thought that men lost their desire due to a sudden loss of testosterone.

New research suggests that men's desire fails due to a gradual fall in testosterone over time. In 2020, the Yale School of Medicine indicated that up to 10-40 percent of adult men have low testosterone, a phenomenon that is increasingly prevalent among young men. A study showed that 20 percent of men aged 15-39 have low levels of testosterone, and because testosterone controls so many body functions, not just sexual, that figure is alarming.

What Women Often Don't Know— Orgasm and the Older Male

Many women I spoke to were surprised to learn that men's orgasms change with age—becoming weaker, less frequent, or disappearing altogether. Desire may remain, but climax doesn't always follow.

Women, by contrast, can experience orgasms well into their eighties.

Sharon described this with wry honesty: her orgasms were so strong they left her exhausted for the rest of the day. Her partner's, when they occurred at all, were barely noticeable.

No one had told her this was normal. If women had known earlier, many said, they would have understood their partners better—and blamed themselves less.

Viagra Fixes Plumbing—Only

When men seek medical help, the solution is often mechanical. Viagra. Cialis. Pills that improve blood flow. They work—sometimes.

But they don't fix desire. They don't address fear. And they certainly don't repair wounded identity.

They are often contraindicated, and doctors are reluctant to prescribe because of the patient's existing medical issues, such as hypertension. Other men bypass doctors entirely, buying pills online, risking their cardiac health rather than admitting vulnerability. Who knows what is in those tablets from China, India, Thailand, Spain or Korea?

The desperation has had bizarre consequences. Powdered rhinoceros horn—long believed to be an aphrodisiac—has contributed to the species' near extinction. It doesn't work, of course. But the myth survives because male anxiety is ancient and lucrative.

Dr Chris Church, a general practitioner of over forty years, shared his thoughts. "I don't think it's loss of masculine identity that diminishes desire, rather a loss of erectile ability causes frustration initially and eventually a sense of the inevitable. Many men are pleasantly surprised but sceptical when it's explained that erection is a vascular event and that smoking, high cholesterol, obesity, sleep apnoea, diabetes, and so on impair arterial (hence erectile) function and that drugs such as Viagra and Cialis can affect erection in many cases. Of course, the underlying issues need to be addressed, as well as non-vascular causes."

He continues, "When Viagra first became available, men were generally too embarrassed to ask for a prescription, let alone present it to the pharmacist. Nowadays, things have changed, and their main concern is the cost," he says.

"Older men often come into the surgery clearly embarrassed and mutter things like, I have a few problems below. Many years ago, when I was in a semi-rural practice, a tall, well-to-do, somewhat weather-beaten farmer, well into his eighties, came to see me with a minor problem. I had the feeling something else was bothering him. On further enquiry, he sheepishly replied that he had been having 'trouble down below, you know, getting it going, and my lady is not happy.' I began to diplomatically explain the issues of erectile function in older age, saying, 'Look, I am sure if you explain what I'm about to say, your wife will understand...'

He interrupted me: 'My wife couldn't care less. It's my lady down the road that's getting upset.'"

Erectile dysfunction is not just an issue for older men. It is increasingly happening to younger men, too. Theories abound as to the reason why. Perhaps it's all the oestrogen in the water from HRT and the pill—that would be women's fault, of course. Some say it's from watching too much porn.

Do older women care that much about a limp penis?

The answer is complicated: yes and no. No, women don't care so much about the man not being able to have an erection, but yes, they do care about how it affects their partner's self-esteem. Women don't usually mourn the loss of erections. They mourn what comes with them: touch, closeness, reassurance.

By contrast, Sharon and her partner talked. They adapted.

They centred her pleasure. The relationship deepened. The difference wasn't anatomy. It was communication.

Susan and her partner were not so lucky. "He became very depressed when his body didn't cooperate with his desires, and there was unquestionable tension between us. We grew distant as he thought I was coming on to him whenever I tried to cuddle him." Susan lost out on the intimacy she craved.

Susan described how her husband's prostate illness slowly dismantled their intimacy. He interpreted cuddling as pressure. She retreated. They slept in the same bed but lived separate emotional lives. They became, she said, "like brother and sister."

In this case, Susan's husband's erectile dysfunction was the first sign of illness. Yet, that is not always the case for other men. According to Dr Spitz, a leading urologist, erectile dysfunction is caused by a disease with no cure: ageing. He states that 40 percent of men will experience some degree of the problem by the age of forty. This percentage goes up with the years, so 50 percent of men have ED by the age of sixty, and so it goes on. Logically, a one hundred year old has no chance. Eventually, the blood vessels that pump up the penis become stiffer, more fragile and narrower. They are a fraction of the size of the coronary arteries that supply the heart. So, the penis is the first to go, well before a heart attack or stroke.

What This Means for Couples

When men lose sexual function, many lose interest altogether. Some women still want intimacy but are too embarrassed to ask. Silence settles in.

And yet, when couples are willing to reimagine sex—beyond performance, beyond penetration—something unexpected can happen.

Sex can become more generous. More attentive. More intimate.

A functioning penis is not the heart of good sex. Connection is. Which brings us to the most important question of all: If men and women change differently—physically, emotionally, sexually—how do couples navigate intimacy together in later life?

That is where we turn next.

VIII

Mind the Gap

"I love Keith. I do; we have been through so much together. But when it comes to sex, there's always this gap. It's not like there's a lack of physical attraction—far from it. It's more like this unspoken chasm."—Wendy, 77

Sex is often described as a shared experience: two people wanting the same thing at the same time, meeting neatly in the middle.

In real life—especially in long relationships—it rarely looks like that.

For many couples, there's an invisible gap. Not always a lack of love. Not even a lack of attraction. More often, it's a mismatch in expectations, timing, confidence, and the meaning each partner attaches to sex. Everyone is trying; nobody feels fully understood; and the subject becomes so loaded it's easier to avoid it altogether.

Wendy put it perfectly: she and Keith weren't lacking chemistry. They were living with an unspoken chasm.

So what creates that gap? And how do couples cross it without turning the bedroom into a negotiation table?

Let's start with the basics—because that's often where misunderstandings begin.

Bodies: Different Equipment, Different Experiences

It sounds obvious, but anatomy matters.

For men, sexual pleasure is concentrated primarily in one visible organ with an impatient timetable. When he was young, he could be aroused quickly, climax quickly, recover quickly—and expect the whole system to behave on demand. So, when the penis fails him later in life, it isn't just inconvenient. It can feel like a personal humiliation.

Women's bodies, on the other hand, are more distributed. Pleasure is not confined to one external switch. It involves the clitoris, the vulva, the vagina, the mind, the mood, and sometimes, if their partner has put the bins out. We also have an unfair advantage: the clitoris has roughly twice as many nerve endings as the penis. We don't mention this to boast. We mention it because it explains why women may enjoy sex in ways that don't rely on penetration—and why "performance" is often a male obsession more than a female one.

Men may be able to orgasm quickly. When they were young, some could do it repeatedly. But biologically, most remain what we might affectionately call one-trick ponies: one ejaculation, and it's lights out, thank you and goodnight.

Women can have multiple orgasms at many ages. The intensity may change over time, but the capacity does not vanish—if the woman wants them, and if the conditions allow.

And that right there is the first gap.

Men may brag about the number of times that they have sex in a night, but who cares? For women, the frequency of sex is not that important. It's the quality. As they say in the trades, quality always supersedes quantity. Women are the show's stars. Sexually, men are in the chorus line.

Hormones: The Drama Queens of Desire

Desire isn't only about anatomy. Hormones matter too. Testosterone influences sexual desire in both men and women, though men have more of it. For many men, this means libido can feel relatively steady for years—until age, stress, illness, or low testosterone changes the equation.

Women's desire is more variable. For decades, it fluctuates with the cycle, pregnancy, exhaustion, emotional load, relationship security, stress, and then menopause. Which means many women recognise themselves in this maddening reality: one day you feel alive and interested; the next you feel like a tired administrator who cannot possibly be expected to add sex to the to-do list. "I'm way too tired for this. I have a headache."

Women's hormones can be an emotional rollercoaster. Men often find this mystifying—until they are on the rollercoaster themselves, in later life, when their own bodies become less reliable.

Orgasm Inequality: When Men Arrive, Women's Pleasure Sometimes Leaves

Now for the most uncomfortable truth.

Heterosexual men tend to orgasm far more frequently during sex than heterosexual women. That difference is so consistent across studies that it has a name: the orgasm gap. Women are completely different. It depends on who they are having sex with!

It's not that women's bodies are "too complicated." It's that women's pleasure has not been prioritised.

Say it out loud: as soon as men enter the picture, women's orgasm rates often drop.

This isn't because men are cruel. It's because many couples have been taught that sex equals penetration and male climax—end of story. Women, taught to be polite and not "make a fuss," go along with it. Men, taught to take pride in being "good in bed," assume everything is fine—especially when women are skilled at acting.

And that creates the second gap:

Men feel they are doing well. A study in the U.S. found that men experience orgasms about 95 percent of the time during sex, while straight women experience orgasms only 40-60 percent of the time.

In contrast, women who have sex with other women experience orgasm 86 percent of the time. So, what's going on here? No penis required, then?

This stark difference suggests that the presence of men seems to be linked to lower orgasm rates for women. Say that again? It looks like as soon as men enter the picture, women's pleasure goes down. Because when women are having sex with themselves, ahem, masturbation, the rate of orgasm is even higher. When women engage in masturbation, their orgasm rate is comparable to men's—over 95 percent.

Women feel they are missing something but don't know how to ask.

The emotional consequences are obvious. Women can feel frustrated, unfulfilled, even disconnected. Men may sense something is off and feel inadequate or guilty. Over time, this can produce resentment, withdrawal, or polite avoidance disguised as "we're just tired."

Throughout time, men have been in the driving seat as far as sex in relationships… except when age lets them down, and that's when they often throw in the towel and withdraw altogether. It can be too painful for them even to discuss it, as Susan tells us. "My husband became very depressed when his body didn't cooperate with his desires, and there was unquestionable tension between us."

Silence took over the space where touch used to be.

Distraction and Desire: Why Women Lose the Thread

Here's another difference many couples recognise instantly.

Women are more easily knocked out of sexual focus by stress and distraction. A baby crying. A parent getting frail. Work worries.

Family dynamics. A barking dog. The memory that you promised to bring something to the grandchildren's school event. Women don't seem to lose that; even grandmothers remain on high alert for babies' cries.

Men—generally—can stay more narrowly focused when aroused.

Men find it easier to block out these distractions and keep their focus on sexual arousal. I don't believe a sexually aroused male responds to a baby's crying quite like the baby's mother.

Whether that's biology, social conditioning, or convenience is up for debate. But it's a real difference in many relationships, and it becomes more pronounced with age as responsibilities and anxieties multiply.

One woman told me her husband confessed to sleeping with a colleague. Her first question was: "Didn't you think of the children?"

We can imagine his thoughts: Not at the precise moment her hand went down my jeans, no.

This is not an excuse. It's a portrait of the gap in how men and women often process consequences—especially in the heat of desire.

The Cultural Double Standard: Men Age, Women Disappear

As if biology weren't enough, culture piles on.

Society expects men to remain sexually active and desirable. Newspapers cheer when elderly men father children. 'Still got lead in the pencil,' they say, as younger men applaud, imagining themselves as future heroes.

We even have the "silver fox" stereotype—George Clooney and his brethren—proof that men can age into attractiveness.

Women, meanwhile, are trained to believe youth equals desirability. Whole shelves of books about "ageing well" for women mostly mean: look younger. If you stay "fresh" you might remain worthy of attention. If you don't, you become invisible.

Gwen made a comment that should be printed on a tea towel and slapped onto billboards:

"There's this feeling we should just be grateful someone still wants to be intimate with us. Women's desires are dismissed or ridiculed. It's like society says, 'Just be grateful, woman, that men still want to have sex with you.'"

Bollocks to that, Gwen added. "Men would have sex with a watermelon if they were desperate enough."

It's vulgar, yes. It's also true enough to make you laugh—and then realise what women have been swallowing for decades.

And here is the third gap:

Men are socially permitted desire. Women are socially punished for it.

The Role of Frequency: Can it Improve Satisfaction?

After a relationship becomes established, it has been reported that many women experience fewer orgasms than men during sex. This can impact their relationship. As Rutgers social psychology student Wetzel explains, if women begin to expect less pleasure, the inequality may persist and even worsen over time.

It's like biting into your favourite chocolate bar and discovering that the manufacturer has changed the formula, and you no longer want to buy it. When women expect less pleasure, it can create a cycle of feeling dissatisfied. Often, men may not realise that their partner isn't delighted and might assume that their sexual experience is similar to their own. We already know that men often struggle to determine whether their partner is faking.

Yet both partners benefit when each person experiences

pleasure. Mark, who shared his story with me, said that he particularly enjoys watching his partner reach orgasm, and sometimes, it is enough for him that he has given her pleasure.

Bridging the Gap: Sandra and David

Sandra and David, both in their seventies, show what happens when people stop performing and start talking.

David, a widower, was hesitant about dating. He had loved his wife. He felt disloyal. And he feared his ageing body would disappoint. Sex, to him, was tied to competence. He was anxious about whether he could "meet expectations," as if intimacy were an exam.

Sandra approached it differently. She was not auditioning for youth. She wanted a connection. She understood that intimacy changes shape as we age, and that tenderness and honesty can be more erotic than perfection.

Over time, they talked. Not in a dramatic way—just steady, human truth-telling about fears, desire, insecurities, and what they actually wanted now.

David began to understand something many men reach too late: intimacy isn't about looking a certain way or performing a certain role. It is about feeling safe and intimacy.

Their relationship became fulfilling not because bodies stayed young, but because they stopped demanding youth from each other.

Navigating the Disconnect: Communication and Understanding

The gap between men and women is not only biology. It is culture. Habit. Shame. Silence. The scripts we inherited and never questioned. But there is good news. The gap is not permanent.

When couples learn each other's realities—anatomy, arousal, desire, fear, pride, tenderness—sex becomes less of a test and more of a conversation. And intimacy becomes something you build, not something you either "have" or "lose."

Which leads to the next question:

If the gap is real—and it is—what are the practical ways couples cross it, especially when bodies change and confidence wobbles?

That is where we go next.

IX

Mission Possible:
Closing the Gap

"I never thought I'd be sitting here talking about the bright pink vibrator in my hand. But here we are. And honestly, I'm not embarrassed."—Anita

At eighty-one, Anita is holding a bright pink vibrator. Not as a joke. Not as a provocation. But as a symbol. Of self-knowledge. Of independence. Of pleasure reclaimed.

She is not ashamed. Why should she be? She understands something many women reach late, if at all: intimacy does not expire. It changes, yes—but it can still surprise, delight, and nourish us if we let it.

This chapter is about how women and couples close the gap— not by trying to be younger, but by being braver.

The Burden of Keeping the Flame Alive

We are told—relentlessly—that keeping a relationship alive depends on sex. And that keeping sex alive depends, somehow, on women.

Magazine covers shout instructions: spice things up, rekindle the spark, be irresistible again. Men's magazines are curiously silent on the matter. The message is unmistakable: if desire fades, it's the woman's fault.

Germaine Greer observed decades ago that equality in relationships would only arrive when women stopped being passive. Despite everything we have gained, many women still carry the emotional labour of intimacy—soothing egos, managing disappointment, pretending satisfaction.

But intimacy is not a solo performance. In reality, intimacy is a shared experience. Men also age. Testosterone drops, health issues arise, and performance often declines—but these challenges are rarely discussed. As therapist Esther Perel points out, many long-term couples face intimacy struggles that affect both partners, not just women.

Bodies falter—confidence wobbles. And yet the burden of adaptation often lands squarely on women's shoulders.

Susan, 63, saw this firsthand. When her husband's body no longer did what he wanted, he withdrew. "There was unquestionably tension between us," she says. The emotional weight of his frustration fell on her shoulders. She carried the emotional fallout.

At this stage of life, many women are done with that. The

burden of keeping the flame alive is not ours alone. Ultimately, relationships flourish when both partners invest in the emotional, physical, and intimate aspects of the bond. It's not one person's job to keep the flame alive. Desire and excitement are mutual responsibilities—and it's time for everyone to recognise that.

When Desire Isn't Dead—Just Bored

Sometimes the gap has nothing to do with illness, hormones, or ageing bodies. Sometimes sex has become dull.

Jane put it bluntly: "I don't want to have sex with a tired older man who does the same thing every time."

She wasn't frigid. She was bored.

Routine kills desire faster than age ever could. When intimacy becomes predictable, mechanical, or joyless, withdrawal is not pathology—it's self-preservation.

The problem is not that women want less sex. It's that they want better sex.

Long Relationships and the Desire Paradox

Wednesday Martin has written that long-term relationships can be particularly tough on female desire—not because women are fickle, but because desire thrives on novelty, curiosity, and imagination. Many women—like those in the Australian film *The Little Death* (2014)—express that it's not just sexual pleasure they crave but a deeper, more meaningful connection that stimulates both their body and mind.

Many women crave not just orgasm, but engagement—being seen, wanted, mentally stirred. But what happens when a partner doesn't understand their needs, and they are in a relationship with a man who can't manoeuvre his way around a roundabout, let alone a clitoris

Heavy-handed partners who received imperfect sex education, such as older men who were teenagers in the sixties, employing the techniques they picked up behind the bike sheds at school, are not likely to understand their partner's needs. Or those who latterly gained their understanding by watching porn. Don't get me started on porn.

Which explains an awkward truth: women labelled "frigid" often rediscover desire the moment a new partner appears. It isn't the woman who was broken. It was the sex.

Films like *Good Luck to You Leo Grande* (2022), give voice to this reality. Emma Thompson's character doesn't want more sex—she wants meaningful, attentive, pleasurable sex. And she refuses to be ashamed of wanting it. Emma commented at the premiere of the film that she didn't think that female pleasure had ever been at the top of the list of things that the world wants to talk about.

Older Women Want—and Deserve—Pleasure

Gwen, eighty-five, met a man during rehabilitation after knee replacements. She was astonished by how much she enjoyed being courted.

"I thought older women were past love and desire," she said. "It's not true."

The myth that women age out of longing is persistent—and wrong.

What changes is not desire itself, but women's tolerance for disappointment.

The Secret Art of Loving an Older Woman

At last, we are admitting to the world and ourselves that getting older doesn't spell the end of a woman's sex life. Some women now want the sex they have been reading about, which they never had in their marriages: sex toys, oral sex, different positions, and much more. Be open; put aside the old ideas you learned from your parents, school, and others, and concentrate on what you truly want.

As one of my friends, who attends the same language course that I do, suggested, "Men should forget learning German and become a cunnilinguist instead." She wasn't joking.

The Stale Marriage—Some Solutions For

Anthropologist Helen Fisher reminds us that novelty fuels desire. New experiences activate the brain's reward systems. Routine dulls them.

Sometimes, novelty is as simple as remembering what first attracted you. A look. A laugh. A uniform.

One TV chef's wife admits she occasionally asks him to wear his chef's jacket to bed. Firefighters. Police officers. Surgeons in scrubs—fantasy has always played a role in desire.

Why should imagination retire?

Love Needs Closeness—Desire Needs Space.

This is the paradox at the heart of long relationships.

Love wants familiarity. Desire wants mystery.

At the beginning of a relationship, there's often this air of mystery. Then we tried to give the illusion that we didn't go to the toilet, fart or have periods; we were fun and undemanding every time we went on a date.

Ours is Not a Farting Relationship

We move in together, abandon illusion, and stop trying. Tatty tracksuits replace allure. Bathroom doors stay open. Romance is postponed indefinitely.

The boomer generation was brought up to keep some things private. However, later generations want to live authentically and honestly. They think keeping bodily functions private is not so necessary. Let it all hang out. When they set up a house together, they feel there is no need to make a big effort for their partners, who may have seen them giving birth or vomiting up a bad curry. They roll around with laughter when we tell them that some of us changed into our nightgowns in the bathroom on the wedding night. So, they wear their tatty tracksuits, reserving makeup and nice clothes for work, not for their partners. They give their partners the scraps

Joan Collins—on her fifth marriage at ninety—swears by separate bathrooms she believes that they are the secret of a long marriage. Considering she is in her fifth marriage and ninety years old, I think her evidence is as credible as that of an academic. She also spends much of the year in France, and French women seldom reveal their entire bodies at once, thereby preserving a sense of mystery and allure. French women preserve mystery by revealing less, not more.

Living Apart, Together—and Other Creative Solutions

Some couples find balance through Living Apart Together relationships—separate homes, shared commitment. Others have separate bedrooms. Many couples in second marriages or long-term partnerships find that the idea of always sharing the same space becomes less appealing over time, so they are exploring living apart together, where they maintain separate living spaces while keeping their relationship intact.

Take Prue Leith, for example, the famed UK chef and television personality who has spoken openly about her relationship. She loves the way her relationship with her husband works: they get all the joy of being together without the daily responsibilities of cohabitation. As she puts it, "What you want—and what I get—is him without his clobber and without the responsibility of looking after his laundry or sewing on his buttons." It's a clever way to maintain love and desire without the burden of daily routines or unspoken expectations.

The Sleep Divorce

If we don't want to live apart, we don't always have to sleep in the same bed.

A sleep divorce doesn't mean a relationship is on the rocks—it simply means that partners sleep in separate beds to improve the quality of their sleep. As we age, sleep quality can become more challenging. One partner might snore, wake up frequently, or have different sleep preferences, making the idea of sharing a bed uncomfortable. A partner switching on the lights and stumbling around is not helpful (that's putting it mildly). If truth be told, it's really annoying. We don't necessarily want to change partners, but having separate bedrooms may actually bring us closer together. After all, the kids have probably left home by now, so some space has been vacated.

Beth's story illustrates this beautifully. Beth's husband, Clive, was a chronic snorer, and after many years of tossing and turning, they both decided that sleeping apart was the solution.

Mornings, once a source of frustration, now felt like a peaceful sanctuary. Beth woke to the quiet of her own bed, free from the noise that had kept her awake for so long. Clive, on the other hand, preferred his military-grade mattress, which suited his disciplined nature, having spent many years in the Royal Marines.

They'd found their own rhythm, a balance that suited their needs, free from the pressure of what marriage should look like. Beth realised that while they may not sleep together, they were still together. And in the end, that was enough.

They were still together—just better rested.

Desire Beyond the Bedroom: Trading Hearts: The Courage to Choose New Love

In the rhythm of love, sometimes it's not about holding on tighter but about letting go and stepping into a new embrace. Changing partners isn't the end—it could be the start of a new chapter, a chance to rediscover yourself and the kind of love you deserve. As Christine and Paul discovered, there is nothing like a change of partner to get the hormones rushing again, but it's not for everyone.

Many women found satisfaction when they changed partners. The Coolidge Effect is a term biologists and psychologists use to describe a behavioural phenomenon common to most mammal species. This need for variety in sexual relationships has been touched on before but let the men and President Coolidge have the last word on this subject.

The President and Mrs Coolidge were on a tour of a chicken farm. Mrs Coolidge commented that one of the roosters was frequently mating. She asked the attendant how often that happened.

"Dozens of times each day", the chicken farm attendant replied.

Mrs Coolidge said, "Tell that to the President when he comes by."

The attendant duly passed this message from his wife to the

President.

To which Coolidge replied, "Same hen every time?"

The reply was, "Oh no, Mr President, a different hen every time."

Coolidge then turned to the attendant and said, "Tell that to Mrs Coolidge!"

Changing partners is not for everyone. But neither is staying where intimacy has died.

Intimacy Beyond Sex

Often, what women miss most is not intercourse—but touch.

As we grow older, we may find that what we truly crave isn't always sex but intimacy. Changing partners can seem like an unnecessary hassle when what we really want is a connection that goes beyond physicality. Many of us have spent years with a partner, training them to handle the "boring" tasks—from taking the car in for service to dealing with things that go bump in the night. So why replace them when what we're really missing is the closeness and comfort of intimacy?

Intimacy is easy to take for granted when it's present, but once it's gone, we often realise just how much we miss it. For many women, it's not the sex itself they miss after being on their own but the warmth and connection that intimacy provides. Sophie, who had been living alone for only a short time, shared how much she missed the frequent, simple touch that had once connected her to her partner.

"It's not the kind of touch you get from a masseur—no matter how skilled they may be. It's the casual, everyday affection we often experience in younger years: a hand on the back, a brush of the arm, the warmth of someone next to you on the couch."

As Gwen put it, "The electrifying thrill of touch doesn't fade; it just becomes more meaningful."

For Suzi, being widowed set her off on a wild, unexpected journey. She discovered something people actually have a name for: Widow's Fire. It's that sudden craving for touch, heat, and yes—lust—that comes roaring back when you least expect it. In the stillness of grief, she found herself missing not just the comfort of a hand to hold, but the spark of desire, the reminder that her body was still very much alive.

Longing for touch is not weakness. It is biology. It is humanity.

What Endures

Of course, intimacy is about more than lust. The real glue in long-term love is the emotional kind—the trust, tenderness, and understanding that grow over time. Psychologist Robert Sternberg refers to it as one side of the "triangle of love," alongside passion and commitment. Without intimacy, even the most faithful partnership can start to feel empty.

But here's the thing: passion and tenderness don't have to disappear with age or loss. They just shift. A hand on the shoulder, a soft kiss, fingers entwined—those little gestures carry both comfort and desire. It's about knowing your partner loves you not only for your body, but for who you are—mind, soul, and yes, skin. As Christine told me,

"When physical intimacy became harder for me, I leaned into the emotional side. But the spark was still there—I wanted the kisses, the closeness, the little moments that kept desire alive."

And that is the point. Closing the gap is not about restoring youth. It is about telling the truth.

About curiosity. About courage. And above all, about refusing to believe that intimacy has an expiry date.

X

Love, Lust and Lies

"It wasn't until I was sixty-five, and had been married forty years, that I had satisfactory sex. Obviously, it wasn't with my husband."—Anon

Some sentences land like a champagne cork to the forehead. You laugh first—because what else can you do?—and then you feel the sting underneath.

That woman wasn't confessing to shock me. She was telling the truth the way older women sometimes do when they've finally run out of patience for pretending. Not bitter. Not dramatic. Just... accurate.

And it made me wonder if we are living too long.

Not in the morbid sense. In the practical sense. Because we are now facing dilemmas our grandmothers barely had time to encounter, decades of life after the children have grown, decades of marriage after the "busy years," decades of bodies changing while the relationship stays locked in the same old choreography.

We promised "until death do us part" as twenty-somethings when death was, statistically speaking, much closer.

The phrase "until death do us part" appeared in the English-speaking world following the first printing of the *Church of England's Book of Common Prayer* in 1549. This was a time long before defibrillators, open-heart surgery, and chemotherapy became standard treatments for our illnesses. People were dying like flies then, and death haunted them every day. Some women living in these bygone times often lost their lives when giving life to a new one. In the 19th and first half of the 20th century, everybody knew about death in childbirth, and maternal deaths were running at about twenty-five in a thousand. Men quickly remarried after the deaths of their wives to provide a mother for their children. They had to return to work to provide for their large families, and there was no social security to prop up the family income. So, monogamy during the last century served a purpose; it was compatible with life, forming a pair bond to raise children. But life and society have changed. Fewer women die in childbirth, and life expectancy has increased. Perhaps it's time to rethink our approach to fidelity.

Monogamy made sense as a social structure when life was short, families were large, women were financially trapped, and survival depended on a pair bond.

But what happens when survival is no longer the main project—yet the vow remains?

The Monogamy Problem Nobody Wants to Admit

Mason Cooley wrote, "Monogamy is like reading the same book over and over."

Some of us would argue back: Yes, but it's your favourite book, and you know where the good bits are.

Others would say: I'm sorry, I've reached the middle chapters, and it's all footnotes and damp dialogue.

The truth is, monogamy has always been a dilemma. We just didn't used to talk about it out loud.

Now we do—sometimes badly, sometimes with the help of celebrities who announce "open marriages" with the casual confidence of people who can afford separate houses and a publicist. The rest of us watch from our modest kitchens and think, Well, if they can, can we? And then we remember the mortgage, the grandkids, and the fact we can barely organise a weekend away without someone turning up in odd shoes.

Still, the question nags:

We know that women's sexual desires sometimes change as they age. A new partner may ignite any dormant sexual passions and give us a new lease of life.

Take Gwen, for instance, in her 1980s, who embarked on an exhilarating sexual affair with a man ten years her junior after having been widowed for many decades of marriage. Though hardly a "toy boy" himself, he stirred a passion in her that he also felt. She never anticipated experiencing such passion again. What surprised her was that she experienced excitement and sexual arousal, just like when she was young. "I have never felt so alive, and I forget about my arthritis."

Those hormones, oxytocin and endorphins, with their pain relieving qualities, had emerged from retirement and were once again working their magic. These feel-good hormones, released during sex, activate the pleasure centres in the brain, creating relaxation and intimacy. Is infidelity the antidote to the monotony of long-term monogamy? Is an affair the answer to the boredom of monogamy?

Do we really expect one person to be everything—lover, confidant, co-parent, companion, nurse, audience—for fifty or sixty years?

The Real Reason Affairs Happen

People like to believe affairs are about sex. Sometimes they are.

Often they aren't.

Affairs are as likely to begin with a feeling as they are with a body: the feeling of being noticed, being desired, being seen again. The feeling of vitality. The feeling of having a self that isn't just "wife," "husband," "mum," "dad," "grandmother," "grandfather," "the one who pays the bills."

One man—Alexander—shocked himself (and thrilled his seventy-year-old lover) when he texted, "I wish I was in bed with you right now."

Who wouldn't feel their pulse jump?

Your partner of forty years is not going to send a message like that during his lunch break. He's more likely to text: Do we have any milk?

That is not a criticism. It's simply what long life together does: it replaces pursuit with practicality. The romance isn't always gone, but the language changes. And when the language of desire disappears, people start to look for it elsewhere.

Let's be honest—infidelity happens. It happens in every culture, in every corner of the world. No amount of fear, guilt, or religious pressure seems strong enough to completely suppress sexual desire or the excitement that can come with breaking the rules.

Despite the taboo, the numbers suggest infidelity is more common than we like to admit. Some studies estimate that about 20 to 30 percent of married couples experience affairs. Psychologist Dr Shirley Glass, who spent years researching this topic, came to a similar conclusion in her book *Not Just Friends*. She argued that infidelity isn't always about sex—it's often about emotional connection, opportunity, or unmet needs.

Then there's Shere Hite, a groundbreaking sex researcher whose work stirred up even more controversy. In *The Hite Report*, published in the 1970s, she suggested that as many as 70–80 percent of people in marriages might be unfaithful in some form. Her research dug deep into emotional dissatisfaction and the complex reality of human intimacy, especially from the perspective of women. Her findings challenged many social norms—and she paid a price. The backlash was so intense that she eventually left the U.S. and disappeared from public life in Europe.

Of course, all this research depends on people being honest. And when it comes to something as personal as infidelity, that's not a given. Some people lie to protect themselves, others to protect their partners—or their image. Who tells the truth when approached by a researcher with a clipboard? So while the exact numbers might be fuzzy, one thing is clear: infidelity is far more common and far more complex than most of us are willing to admit.

Why Does an Affair Happen?

There are a hundred theories on why people have affairs. Psychologists give us some ideas and describe psychological, sociological and economic reasons contributing to infidelity. It could be as simple as being too busy for each other and searching for new partners to fit into a world that tells us we must have a great sex life to be happy and fulfilled. Others want to escape the boredom and chase the thrill of being desired.

Researchers and therapists offer lists of reasons—anger, neglect, low commitment, need for variety, loneliness, opportunity. But the stories I heard circled one truth again and again:

Most affairs were not about mind-blowing sex. They were about wanting to touch and be touched—without being invisible.

As Esther Perel puts it, affairs often aren't a search for another person so much as a search for another self.

What Counts as an Affair, Anyway?

This is where things get messy. Is it an affair if there's no sex?

What about flirting? Sexting? An ongoing emotional confidante? Porn? A hotel-room massage on a boys' trip? A one-night stand at a conference? Falling in love?

President Clinton famously insisted he "did not have sexual relations with that woman," which did nothing to clarify the definition, but did introduce the world to a lot of creative parsing.

Here's a simpler test: if it's a secret, and it would wound your partner if they knew, it has crossed a line.

Affairs thrive on secrecy. And secrets always cost someone. Usually, it's the spouse who pays first—often the woman—and not always because of the sex.

Heather, who discovered racy texts her husband had sent, said something I heard repeatedly:

"It wasn't the sexual betrayal that destroyed me. It was the emotional part. I knew he was in love with her."

That's the cruel twist. People begin affairs, insisting it's "only physical," "just a bit of fun," "a separate compartment."

Despite all the promises at the beginning of an affair that it will be only physical, only sex, it won't. Because people inevitably fall in love. Falling in love ended Pamela's experience with partner swapping when she was much younger. It was very exciting, but it became serious, so it had to come to an end.

It seems particularly unfair for women, but it is just how it is. We can blame chemistry. The hormones released during sex, namely oxytocin, work their biochemical magic and enable us to fall in love, whether we like it or not. These hormones are our pleasure. They are also our downfall. These cunning little neurotransmitters are intimately related to stimulating the mind's pleasure centres, allowing us to slip easily and inevitably into bonding and care. Why? It's because that's the way it is. Nature has its agenda. Physical closeness produces dopamine and serotonin. We call that love. That is one of the dangers of open marriages; it is lovely to have extra-marital sex, but then one of the partners falls in love and spoils everything. They start exchanging confusing emails, declaring, 'I love my life, I love where I live, I love my kids, and I love my dog, and yet I love you as well.'

Why Affairs Feel Like Magic

Affairs are intoxicating because they are free of domestic reality.

No dentist appointments. No council rates. No wet towels on

the bed. No arguments about money. No adult children ringing at inconvenient times. No one is loading the dishwasher while the other asks, "Have you seen my glasses?"

Affairs are all champagne and possibility. They are a holiday from the monotony of life.

And then they end.

Jenny, who had lived through it, described the aftermath with brutal honesty: you're shattered for a while, and then— eventually—you stop giving a fuck, and it's the best feeling ever.

There is no shortcut through heartbreak. You endure it until you don't.

Therefore, there are many reasons to seek solace outside a committed relationship, and just as many reasons not to.

Sex therapists will tell us that an affair may be less spontaneous and perhaps the first step out of a relationship a person has already decided to leave—emotionally, if not physically. It's not generally acknowledged, but it's believed that even in a committed relationship, many people have someone in mind, almost in cold storage, on standby if or when their current relationship ends. They might not overtly think about it, but they have an affair because they need something in place before ending their current relationship, someone perhaps who loved them before or is in their life now as a friend. Is it a coincidence that many older couples find love together with someone who has been in their friendship circle when they were young? After a temperate marriage, Lorna found love with an old school friend she had dated in her teenage years.

Sometimes It Isn't About Sex—It's About Being Alive.

Gwen—yes, Gwen again, because Gwen is proof that the human heart never retires—had an affair with a married man. She did not try to dress it up as noble.

"It wasn't so much about the sex," she said. "It was intimacy. Connection. I felt alive. And it's wonderful to be desired."

Jenny described her emotional affair the same way. She was drowning in the demands of young children and ageing parents, trapped in a life that felt like duty without joy. The man she leaned on didn't rescue her—he reminded her she existed.

Tony explained his infidelity, which escalated into an intense love affair that nearly destroyed his marriage and that of his lover.

His reason? It was quite simple: "She made me feel important." He stopped short of destroying his marriage by ending the affair, even though he longed to be with his lover. In one of his final messages to his lover, he enclosed an old photograph, taken many years before their affair, of both families at a beachside picnic. Children, dogs, and their respective partners are happy being together. Beneath it he wrote words that were both noble and devastating:

"This is why we could never make a life together. We can't roll back the years. We have what we have: extraordinary memories, and the reassurance that nothing has been lost."

An affair, in these cases, functioned like oxygen. That doesn't make it harmless. It makes it human.

And Sometimes It Really Is About Sex

Some people are in sexless marriages for years. One partner shuts up shop; the other is expected to accept celibacy until death. Why are we so judgmental about that?

If someone doesn't want sex anymore, does that mean their partner must live without touch for the rest of their life? This is the moral knot we don't like to untangle, because it forces us to admit that love, loyalty, and desire are not always neat companions.

The Aftermath: What Happens When the Secret Escapes

Well, obviously, all hell breaks loose, but one thing is sure—nothing will ever be the same again for everyone. The spouse, the lover, and the partners will all be inexplicably changed, leaving irreparable scars on everyone. The fallout is inevitable as it is agonising. Despite all the damage to his marriage and that of his lover, Tony wrote in his farewell letter to her, "I can never go back to how it was; you are part of my DNA."

Something in the atmosphere changes. Trust becomes a haunted house: you can still live in it, but you never quite forget where the floorboards creak.

Heather collapsed into a depression that lasted months. Friends urged medical tests, convinced she was physically ill, because grief can look like disease.

She found a note in her husband's diary—words of longing intended for someone else. That was the part that destroyed her: not the mechanics of sex, but the evidence of emotional replacement.

She was less upset by the sexual betrayal but distraught that he had fallen in love. The words that upset her so much?, "You are my first thought every morning upon waking. I long for the day I wake up and find you still asleep on my shoulder."

Heather said that she and her husband had sex, but not in the way he wanted; he wanted to make love whilst she wanted to get it over and done with.

Affairs are not always the cause of relationship problems. Often they are the symptom—the final leak in a dam that has been quietly cracking for years.

Masculinity, Ego, and the Need to Feel "Enough"

We are quick to condemn men's infidelity (and often rightly), but we rarely examine what some men are actually chasing: not youth, not bodies, but relief from shame.

Tony's story stayed with me because it revealed something tender and ugly at once. It may be that a heterosexual man's ego and identity can be shaken without us even noticing.

He had married the cleverest woman in his university class—a brilliant woman who won prizes and prestige in a world that still didn't expect women to dominate. He admired her. He loved her. He also lived in her shadow.

At a gala dinner where she was the keynote speaker, her place card read: Professor Kenton. His read: Mrs Kenton.

The organisers assumed the important person was male. The companion, female. Everyone laughed. Tony laughed too. He told the story many times.

But beneath the laughter was a wound. A small, sharp humiliation that confirmed a fear he had carried for decades: I am not the important one.

He didn't have an affair because he was sex mad. He had an affair because someone made him feel whole.

"She made me feel important," he said.

Masculine identity is a fragile thing—hard-won, easily lost. We speak readily of men's aggression, but rarely of their identity, of how delicate it is to build and how easily it can be undone. For Tony, his affair was never about the sex. What drew him to his lover was the balm she offered: the assurance that, to her, he was whole, perfect, enough. She gave him back the man he longed to believe he was. He fell in love because she restored what he thought he had lost. And though Tony and his wife soldiered on, stoic as ever, a part of him never stopped remembering the one woman who made him feel complete.

That is the strange thing about affairs: even when they don't destroy a marriage, they change the people inside it.

Infidelity is Not Exclusive to Heterosexual Couples

The eighty-year-old British actor Miriam Margolyes tells an amusing story. "I really fell in love with this woman, and we had a sort of affair, then she fell in love with another actress, and I went crackers, and beat her up and trashed her room, and wrote 'you lesbian cunt' on the mirror, and I was asked to leave."

But when she found herself in an adulterous affair many years later, while in a committed relationship of many years standing, she was distraught. She describes the discovery and aftermath as the worst six months of her life. She had forgotten how strong sexual passion could be. She is ashamed of that painful part of her life but shows courage in her willingness to show her vulnerability by discussing this catastrophic period. She concludes that, 'Adultery is a foolish thing.'

Love, Lust... and the Lies We Tell Ourselves

We also lie in more ordinary ways.

"I love her, but I'm not in love with her," people say—usually after they've left their partner for someone who resembles the partner, just newer packaging.

At the beginning, romantic love is a kind of spell. Psychologists call it limerence. It hijacks the brain, floods the body with chemicals, and makes even the dullest man seem fascinating because he knows how to text properly.

You can't eat. You can't sleep. Nobody is taking the bins out. The world narrows to one person.

It doesn't last. It can't. If it did, civilisation would collapse under the weight of neglected laundry.

After months—sometimes two years—the fog clears. Reality returns. People blame marriage. Or boredom. Or ageing. And then they chase the chemical high again, mistaking the end of infatuation for the end of love.

So... Should We Judge?

Here is the uncomfortable truth I have learned from listening to older women: Affairs are not glamorous. They are not simple. They are not "just sex."

And they are never consequence-free. They expose need. Loneliness. Pride. Neglect. Desire. The ache to feel visible.

None of this excuses betrayal. But it does invite something we don't offer enough in this territory: complexity.

In a world where companionship competes with tradition, where bodies change but longing persists, perhaps our task is not to sneer.

Perhaps it is to look closely—at love, at identity, at the ways we cope with time—and ask better questions than "Who's to blame?"

Because the older we get, the clearer it becomes:

Love is not a single story. It is a library of them.

And some of the chapters are messy.

XI

Divorce, Death
and Dating

"There's no one as optimistic as a woman with a long-term, happy relationship to her name. Of course, I want a partner again. And of course I want sex."

If you ever want proof that the human heart is gloriously unreasonable, look at a woman who's been through the wringer and still says, without apology, Right then—what's next?

Because after divorce or death, we don't just lose a person. We lose a pattern. A home base. A history. The shared language of "remember when". And then we find ourselves, blinking, back at the beginning—standing at the edge of the dating pool with our toes curled, wondering what on earth we are doing.

And here's the first rule of later-life romance:

When you go fishing in the dating pool and land a big fish, it doesn't matter whether he's divorced or widowed—he will come with baggage.

It's never a neat little overnight bag, either. It's the full Samsonite set.

The Baggage: Two Kinds of Past

Men tend to talk about their former partners in one of two ways.

If he is divorced. Either she was the biggest bitch in Christendom, a woman who apparently spent thirty years ruining his life for sport…

… or if she has died, she was a sweet, precious angel whose memory now floats around your relationship like a third presence, smiling beatifically while you try to flirt.

No one wants a ménage à trois with a ghost—especially a saintly one—yet many of us end up there. Sometimes it works.

Sharon found happiness in her new partner partly because he had loved his late wife well. He wasn't stuck in the past; he simply knew what good love looked like, and he wanted it again.

Sometimes it doesn't. Abigail tried with Angus, but she always felt measured against the first wife—her cooking, her humour, her halo. Abigail left, not because she lacked love, but because she could never quite breathe in a room that was already occupied.

Grief doesn't always end when the funeral is over. Sometimes it moves in with you.

Why Widowers Move On So Quickly

Widowers often enter new relationships sooner than widows. This can offend people, particularly adult children, who seem to believe their father should spend the rest of his life loyally staring at a framed photograph and eating beans on toast in silence.

But there are reasons, and they're not always sleazy.

In many cultures, a widower is actively "re-homed" by the community. Rachel told me that in her Jewish circle, the community may find a new wife for a widower within months, and nobody blinks. Part of this is practical.

Historically, men remarried quickly because they needed someone to keep the household running and to look after children while they returned to work. Before social welfare, survival often required a woman's labour. In modern life, it's about loneliness and… laundry and food that doesn't come from a packet. And part of it is emotional.

Women often have deeper friendship networks. Men, particularly of older generations, may have built their emotional life almost entirely inside the marriage. When the wife dies, they lose their confidante, social organiser, and daily companion in one hit. So they reach for a new anchor.

Women and Men: Different Languages of Love

Women often show love through words and emotional expression.

Men, especially older men, tend to show love by doing stuff. Fixing things. Organising things. Building the shed. Bringing you a cup of tea you didn't ask for, precisely the way you like it, while pretending it's nothing.

So here's my blunt (and deeply unromantic) test of whether a widower is ready:

If he has removed his wedding ring, packed away the photos, scattered the ashes, and introduced you to his friends as his girlfriend—he is ready.

This is not poetry. But it is evidence.

Almost a Widow

Death is a clean ending, at least on paper. Illness is not.

Many people live in a halfway house: married, but not to the person they married. Their partner is physically present, but the mind has drifted elsewhere—into dementia, delirium, or the slow disappearance that certain diseases bring.

It is one of the loneliest experiences on earth: being loyal to someone who no longer knows you exist.

Helen pushes her husband's wheelchair along Balmoral Beach. They can't go far. Their life is measured in metres. Their home has quietly transformed into a hospital—hoists, commodes, incontinence pads, disability aids. No one ever asked Helen to become a carer. It simply crept up on her, one small compromise at a time, until her marriage was mostly care.

Can we condemn a marriage devoid of intimacy, plagued by illness, stripped of companionship?

Should we judge if one person seeks solace outside its bounds? I used to think I knew the answer. Now I'm not so sure.

Because unless you have money, or die quickly of a heart attack, or get run over by a bus (which is not the retirement plan we recommend), someone you love will be your carer—or you will be theirs.

And it is brutally lonely.

One dementia nurse and professor put it plainly: she had "absolute sympathy" for people in that situation. It's human instinct to crave companionship. Many people have strong opinions—until it happens to them.

I ran a carers' group at Hornsby Hospital when my father

was a patient. In the time I was there, more carers died than their loved ones. That's not a statistic. It's a warning.

But life is strange. Love blossoms in places it has no business blooming. I saw two carers fall in love right under everyone's noses. After their spouses died, they set up home together. It shouldn't have worked. It did.

Sometimes, the best people are right under your nose.

Peter, Rosemary, and the Sunday Lunch Police

Peter felt cheated. Retirement, he thought, would be the best time of their lives. Retirement had freed him of life's tedious side, such as earning a living, and he imagined that he and his wife would travel and indulge their grandchildren with the available spare cash.

More travel. More grandchildren. More ease.

Instead, his wife slipped into dementia. The wife he had loved became a woman who no longer knew him. He became a visitor in his own marriage.

He kept himself busy. He started learning French and longed to visit Paris. He was pining for another companion.

Loneliness, he discovered, is not so much the absence of people as the absence of "someone to do nothing with". Eventually, he sold the sprawling five-bedroom fortress on Sydney's North Shore and moved into a manageable harbourside apartment with Rosemary—a widow he'd known since primary school.

His children were horrified. They saw betrayal. Disloyalty. A sin.

They offered Sunday lunch as if that should be enough. Peter, bless him, pointed out the obvious: there are still six other days to fill.

He continued visiting his wife daily until the day she died. In the nursing home, she mistook him for a carer. He kept showing up anyway.

Meanwhile, he built a life with Rosemary. They shared friends, Beatles songs, and the sacred 6 p.m. ritual of gin, tonic, and "nibbly bits".

After learning French for several years. he went to Paris at last, at the age of eighty-eight. She was eighty-nine. The neighbours now call him her toy boy.

And the neighbours approve. Naturally.

Widowhood: When the World Goes Quiet

Louise's husband died of multiple myeloma in her early sixties. At first, friends rallied. There were meals, sympathy, and help with the practicalities.

Then the visits slowed. The phone rang less. Real life resumed for everyone else.

That's when Louise discovered what grief really removes.

Not only love. Not only the future. But touch.

"I missed the comfort of a warm body next to mine," she said. "My family bought me a kitten. Lovely gesture—but I wasn't going to get intimacy from a cat, for God's sake."

This is the scandal nobody talks about: grief does not switch off sexuality.

Desire doesn't die because someone else did.

It pauses. It stutters. It returns at inconvenient moments with no regard for social expectations.

And when widows talk about that longing, people act as though they are doing grief wrong—too soon, too eager, too alive.

As if mourning requires celibacy.

As if the only acceptable widow is one who quietly fades into beige. Dammit, no.

As Prue Leith and others agree, love knows no bounds, regardless of age. The well-known star of the *British Bake-Off* series is eighty three years old and currently married to her second husband, seven years her junior at seventy five. She says that falling in love again gives you the dopamine hit your body craves. She described falling in love again at seventy seven:

"It's surprising how you can behave like a sixteen-year-old man in your sixties or a seveteen-year-old in your seventies. You know, it's precisely the same. You fall in love with somebody; you start worrying about why the phone is not ringing and thinking, Can I ring him?

The Point of All This

Later-life love is not tidy.

It's complicated by ghosts—some bitter, some angelic. It's complicated by adult children who want their parents to remain frozen in time. It's complicated by illness, caregiving, loneliness, and the stubborn human need for warmth and belonging.

But it also contains something magnificent:

Even after loss, we still want connection. We still want touch. We still want to be seen.

And if anyone finds that shocking, I suggest they take it up with biology.

XII

Navigating Love and Loneliness

"We aren't supposed to articulate our pleasure; nice girls don't." —Sally Phillips

Joan Baez once sang, Where have all the young men gone? She was singing about war, but she might as well have been describing the dating landscape for older women.

Men die younger than women. That's the mathematics. The rest is culture.

Single older men—divorced and widowed—often seek younger women. It's become a grim little cliché that older men are searching for "a nurse or a purse": someone to look after them, or someone to fund them. And what does that leave women?

Often: each other, our friends, our children, our routines, our resilience—and a long stretch of time where the bed is cold.

It's a fact: many women will be on their own for a large proportion of their lives. When partners leave through death or divorce, the hole is so enormous that some women withdraw entirely. Others fling themselves into busyness and become Super Granny, bridge fiend, golf addict, grey nomad, or knit jackets for distressed penguins.

Anything to avoid the quiet. But the need for warmth doesn't disappear. In fact, it often grows louder.

Adjusting Expectations Without Settling

Here's the tricky balance: with fewer men available, we may need to adjust our expectations. That does not mean settling for rubbish. It means getting realistic about what matters.

In our twenties, we often wanted tall, dashing, clever, and financially secure. Ideally, with a fit body and a future.

In our seventies, the list changes.

Alice—divorced from a high-flying banker—fell in love with a kindly farmer.

"I wouldn't have looked twice at him at university," she said. "He wasn't dashing. But now I want kindness and companionship."

This is not romance declining. It is a romance evolving.

Some women strike gold and find a new partner, often someone they've known all their lives. Suzi and Richard had known each other for years, often vacationing together with their respective partners, and had formed a close-knit foursome. After the loss of their partners, their bond deepened, and what had once been a strong friendship blossomed into love. They eventually decided to live together, finding comfort and companionship in one another after their shared loss.

Because as we age, the question becomes less: Will he sweep me off my feet?

And more: Will he be gentle with my heart?

Adventure: Not Always Sensible, Often Necessary

We can't be too fussy. As Joan Rivers once said, "Honey, he's got a pulse, he's upright—bring him to the party!"

And some women want a little adventure. It's not a moral failure.

Sex work is the oldest profession and has served men well for centuries—it is even mentioned in the Bible. But what of women? Is what is good for the goose good for the gander? Is it our time now to pay for sex and companionship? Male escorts have begun appearing in ads offering their services as massage therapists, with extras (if you ask nicely).

Many women who respond to these ads earn good incomes but don't have the time or appetite for a stable relationship. Recently, on the SBS *Insight* program, a woman openly discussed her weekly engagement with a rent boy. Even more enlightening were a male sex worker's comments to the studio audience. He said

"It's not so much the sex these women want. They crave intimacy and want to touch another human being, maybe in the arms of a safe, reputable male escort. Where's the harm if he is polite, affectionate, and looks good?"

Not thrill. Not a scandal. Touch.

Holiday Romance and the Myth of the Foolish Older Woman

We've all heard the stories, usually told with a smirk.

An older woman goes to a sun-soaked place—The Gambia, Barbados, Bali—meets a young man who calls her "princess," and before long she's glowing with late-life romance... until the visa comes through and he disappears.

People love these stories because they confirm a sneery narrative: older women are desperate, gullible, ridiculous.

But behind the gossip is a far more universal truth: the hunger to be seen, desired, chosen.

Love—or the illusion of it—turns clever people into idiots of all ages. If you think you'd be immune, you haven't been lonely enough yet.

If Porn Is Education, We're All in Trouble

Some women wonder if porn can help, and here we need a clear distinction:

Not the porn men watch. No. No. No.

Male-gaze porn is often about bodies, power, and performance. It tends to treat women as props, not people. Many women find it actively off-putting, because it often has nothing to do with pleasure, tenderness, or reality.

Cindy Gallop put it neatly: sex is about people; porn is about bodies.

Female creators are trying to shift this—porn or erotica made with consent, realism, mutual pleasure, and actual female desire in mind. The hope is not only that women might enjoy it, but that young men might learn what school still fails to teach: women are not slot machines. They do not light up when you insert a penis.

Real women don't come pre-hairless with neat labia and a script. They don't scream in ecstasy at the sight of an erection. And most do not want roughness or anal sex as a default setting.

If porn becomes the main sex educator, we will keep producing men who can locate a remote control in the dark but cannot find a clitoris with a head torch and a map.

Whether we date, remarry, have affairs, take lovers, buy a vibrator, hire an escort, watch erotica, or decide we can't be bothered with any of it—there is one point I want older women to take to bed with them (alone or otherwise):

We are allowed to want what we want.

We are not apologising for wrinkles, opinions, fat bums, dodgy knees, or active imaginations. We are not finishing our lives as a footnote.

We are women. We are alive. And we are wonderful for our age.

XIII

Embracing Love and Intimacy in Aged Care

> ## "The desire for intimacy does not decrease with age, and there is no age at which intimacy—including physical intimacy—is inappropriate."—Dr Daniel Kaplan

Julie Bates works in aged care. She isn't a nurse, a doctor, or a care assistant.

She's a sex worker.

Before anyone clutches their pearls, let's be clear: Julie is not an outlier. Her services—and those of professionals like her—are increasingly being integrated into mainstream aged-care settings. In some facilities, comprehensive care plans now explicitly include guidelines for residents receiving visits from sexual partners, including paid professionals. Nursing staff are not merely tolerant; many are quietly supportive.

As Lyndell Cohen, Care Service Manager at Uniting Care NSW, puts it simply: "We don't have any right to judge them. They never stop feeling."

And that, really, is the heart of it.

Yet society still struggles mightily with the idea that older people—particularly those in aged care—might want, enjoy, or seek intimacy. The very notion provokes embarrassment, ridicule, and sometimes outright disgust. We recoil at the thought of "oldies having sex", as though desire should come with an expiry date stamped somewhere around retirement.

No one wants to imagine older people having sex—except older people.

Who Owns Intimacy?

Sex, intimacy, and desire are relentlessly framed as the property of the young. Youth is marketed as sexy; ageing is not. Yet young people do not have a monopoly on touch, affection, or pleasure— however fiercely they may believe they do.

In aged-care facilities, staff often report that the greatest barrier to residents having a sex life is not physical limitation or cognitive decline, but family interference. Adult children, it seems, appoint themselves gatekeepers of their parents' sexuality.

This should surprise no one. These are, after all, the very same people who once enforced curfews, moralised about teenage behaviour, and panicked over closed bedroom doors.

Still, the discomfort runs deep.

Children do not like thinking about sex and their parents in the same sentence.

Sally married her husband in 1966, when premarital sex was frowned upon and the wedding night was officially—at least in theory—the first time a couple slept together. Her parents would never have allowed her boyfriend to stay the night.

Decades later, when Sally invited her adult children to her wedding anniversary celebration, their reaction was unexpectedly horrified. "Mum," they said, visibly squirming, "we'll come to the party—but please don't make us celebrate the night you first had sex with Dad."

Sally had never thought of her anniversary that way. To her, it marked endurance, companionship, and shared history. To her children, it conjured images they desperately wished to avoid. And that's the point.

Taboos around sex between people who share DNA are part of the universe's grand design. We are not meant to imagine our parents as sexual beings. We prefer them wrapped in cardigans, watching Downton Abbey, sipping tea—not watching something racy, and certainly not discovering pornography.

But denial doesn't make desire disappear.

Time to Bring Back the Condom

This new openness around later-life intimacy brings with it an unexpected problem.

The Baby Boomer generation—those now filling aged-care facilities—came of age during the sexual revolution. They are the free-love generation, and they have not quietly packed that away with their flared trousers and protest banners.

As sexual activity among older adults increases, so too does something no one predicted: sexually transmitted infections.

One of the fastest-growing medical issues in Australian nursing homes is chlamydia, genital herpes, and other STIs previously associated with younger people. Cases among those over 65 have more than doubled in the past decade.

Once upon a time, condoms were about preventing pregnancy. Now, they're about preventing disease. And many older adults simply aren't using them.

What's Driving the Rise?

More Australians over sixty are dating, remarrying, or forming new relationships after divorce or bereavement. Many feel liberated—finally free of pregnancy worries, expectations, and old scripts.

What's missing is education.

Safe-sex messaging largely ignores older adults, leaving many unaware that STIs don't politely bow out at menopause. Untreated infections like syphilis and HIV can be especially dangerous in later life, when the immune system is less resilient.

Public-health campaigns have begun experimenting with creative approaches. In the UK, the relationship charity Relate placed vegetable-themed condom packets among seed displays in garden centres—aubergines, zucchinis, avocados—aimed squarely at retired gardeners enjoying a little greenhouse romance.

Apparently, we're not just living for the three Gs anymore: grandchildren, golf, and gardening. Some of us are gardening sexily.

Welcome to the New Intimacy

If sex can—and does—continue until we finally fall off the perch, then society must find a way to accommodate it with dignity.

The media still shies away from geriatric sex, but cracks are appearing. Jane Fonda and Lily Tomlin's Grace and Frankie brought vibrators for older women into mainstream television. Conversations once whispered are now, tentatively, being aired.

The generation that marched, protested, and reinvented sex

in the 1960s has grown old. Their bodies have changed, but their expectations—and desires—have not evaporated.

Being open to senior sexuality means accepting a simple truth: while bodies age, the need for touch, affection, and pleasure does not.

This change won't happen overnight. Jokes about older women and sex will still echo through RSL clubs, delivered by tired comedians who think shock equals humour.

So let's share one ourselves:

An elderly widower moves into a retirement village and attends the welcome party. "George," the hostess asks, "where were you living before coming to Shady Palms?" "Well," George replies, "I was in jail for murdering my wife." "Oh," says the hostess brightly. "So—you're single then?"

As we navigate this new territory, we might as well do it with humour.

But more than that—with empathy, respect, and an unwavering commitment to human dignity. Because people never stop feeling.

And love, in all its forms, does not retire.

Watch out, world. We older women are here. We are real. We are living among you, and some of us are closer than you think.

XIV

Conclusion: Still Here. Still Wanting. Still Ourselves.

The great secret that all older people share is that you really haven't changed in seventy or eighty years. Your body changes, but you don't change at all."—Doris Lessing

And isn't that the truth? Inside, we're still the same spirited women who wore black eyeliner, pale lips, kinky boots, slept with our boyfriends, and maybe smoked a little something we shouldn't have.

The world has loosened up a lot in the last fifty years. We've watched the fight for gay rights, the rise of feminism, the celebration of transgender identities, and the growing acceptance of love in all its beautiful, messy forms. But here's the odd thing: when it comes to talking about sex and older people—especially older women—the silence has been deafening. Society would have us believe that desire should quietly pack its bags and leave once we hit sixty. What nonsense

We were the first to take the pill, the first to take HRT and now the first to tell the world that we are not done yet with sex and life. We never expected to live this long, but now we are dealing with the aspects of change that living this long presents, particularly where sex is involved. Yes, our bodies have shifted, but our need for intimacy, connection, and pleasure is still very much alive.

We've lived through menopause, divorce, widowhood, and raising children who now tell us what to eat and how to live. And still, here we are—still hungry for connection, for love, for touch, and for intimacy that makes us feel alive.

If there is one thing this book has tried to say—sometimes gently, sometimes bluntly—it is this: desire does not have an expiry date.

We do not stop wanting intimacy because we grow older. We stop talking about it because the world becomes uncomfortable when we refuse to fade quietly into the background. Older women are expected to be grateful, restrained, and discreet. Across these pages, women have spoken honestly—often for the first time—about sex, love, loss, betrayal, grief, boredom, delight, embarrassment, and joy. Some found fulfilment late in life, others lost it and mourned it deeply. Some stayed, some left, some strayed, some reinvented themselves entirely. There was no single right way to live a sexual life—only the courage to acknowledge that it mattered.

What emerges, again and again, is not scandal or excess, but dignity. The dignity of wanting to feel desired. The dignity of needing touch. The dignity of choosing solitude—or adventure—or compromise—or joy. And the dignity of saying, at last, this part of me still counts.

We have lived long enough to know that relationships are complicated, that bodies change, that love does not follow tidy rules. We understand that intimacy is not only about penetration or performance, but about kindness, curiosity, generosity, humour, and presence. Sometimes it is about sex. Sometimes it is about lying beside someone and feeling less alone. Sometimes it is about choosing yourself.

If the youngsters roll their eyes or say "yuck"—let them. They'll get here soon enough, and when they do, they'll thank us for breaking the silence. Because claiming our sexuality, our right to be heard, and our right to pleasure at any age isn't just about us—it's a gift we are leaving to them.

So let's stop treating older women's sexuality as a taboo and start celebrating it. Let's own our stories, share our laughter, and refuse to shrink ourselves to fit outdated expectations.

XV

Stories That Have Never Been Told Before

Maria Rosa, [age 89 ¾ years]: My Neighbours Would be Shocked

So, Maria Rosa, you have a big birthday coming up, you will be ninety in June. Can you tell me what it was like for you growing up as a girl in New South Wales?

I went to a boarding school convent run by nuns when I was ten. The nuns never spoke of sex or periods at all. The girls never talked about such things, even in the dormitory at night. It was taboo. Being in a boarding school, my mother and I exchanged letters, and the nuns read my letters and those my mother sent me. So, when I had my periods and needed more pads, I would write at the bottom of the letter. "PS How is Mary?" That was our code.

Mum died in 1949, so this must have been between 1944 and 1949. In the Catholic church, this is how it was. Girls weren't considered worthy of doing the same things that boys could. For example, there were altar boys and altar girls; the altar boys could be on the altar, but the altar girls could not. We had Mass every morning and had to stay behind the altar because we might be having our periods and would be considered unclean. That was the rule: no women were on the altar. We didn't think about it at the time; culturally, that was the way it was.

How did you feel about that, Maria Rosa?

It was just the way it was. Family life revolved around the father being the head of the family, the breadwinner, and the wife staying home and raising the family. Motherhood was the only option at that time, but I trained as a nurse. So, after I married and went to work at the local hospital, my husband wasn't happy because he felt it would look like he couldn't support me. He wanted me to use my maiden name at work. In those days, the man was supposed to be the breadwinner, so it was embarrassing for him for me to work at the hospital.

What was your sex education like in a convent in the 1930s?

As I said, it was an all-girls school; they call them single-sex schools now, I think. Did I mention that it was Catholic? I was at the Cathedral School and sang in the cathedral choir. There were boys in the choir from the Marist School, too, but we were not allowed to talk to them. We would pass notes along the pews to the boys we liked, and they would write back, so that's how we conversed. Every term, the nuns would take us to the river on a picnic, but we were not allowed to strip and swim. The nuns would be patrolling up and down, and when they passed by us, we would jump in the river for a dip. The next day, the nuns would say, "Stand up all those who went swimming yesterday." So, we would all stand up except for one or two who didn't go in because they had their period. And in those days, you couldn't swim if you had your period, which would go on for a week or so. I don't remember discussing periods ever, even with your mother and especially not with your brothers or father. They would never have had any clue about periods. I had no idea of sex or even how my body worked; my husband was a Catholic and went to a well-known religious school, so we were both ignorant. Before getting married, I was training to be a nurse, and I went out for two years with a medical student. He was Catholic, too, but we never had sex. That was the way it was in those days. We used to kiss and cuddle under the rotunda at the hospital, and when we heard someone going by, we would cough to let them know we were there.

As Catholics, we were told that having intercourse before marriage was a mortal sin; if you died having committed a mortal sin, you would go straight to hell. So, we would have to go to the priest, confess our sins, and receive absolution if we wanted to go to Heaven. Artificial contraception was also a mortal sin, even if you were married. When the pill became available to married women, it was banned by the Catholic Church. In the parish church I attended, when you went up to the altar rail to receive communion, if the priest knew you were taking the pill, he would refuse to give it to you because you were in a state of sin. If I remember correctly, a Dominican priest and a journalist wrote about contraception in the Sydney Morning Herald. The rhythm method was the only approved contraception method, meaning you had to abstain from sex when ovulating. The trouble is that I, like many women, didn't have a regular twenty-eight-day cycle, so we had no idea when we were ovulating. Even as a married woman and a nurse, I didn't understand how I could get this to work for me, and I couldn't ask my celibate priest, who knew even less. We were told to live like brother and sister, with no sex. We had four children. Purgatory existed then, too, but that was where you went if you had committed little sins. If our friends got married, they would have to leave because you couldn't be married in nurse training. Masturbation was also a mortal sin, although I am sure many boys did it. I don't think my children would understand this; all my grandchildren, most of them, have had sex before marriage.

I have never discussed sex with them. I said something once, but my son told me, "Too much information, Mum."

Do you have any thoughts on that? What have you learnt over the years? Have the younger generations missed something by all this jumping into bed?

About sex, you mean? What I learnt now, in my later years, is that when you have intercourse with someone you love, it's more than intimacy. It's pure love; you are truly making love. When you orgasm together, the love and sex are on another level. We don't understand lovemaking. Many men, and I am generalising here, have no idea. Yet sex is all about men and nothing about women. In my generation, we never knew that women had orgasms.

So how did you find out? When did you find out?

It may sound strange to tell you this, but a movie was showing then; it must have been at the Orpheum. My husband wouldn't come, so this must have been forty years ago, but the film was about women orgasming. Remember, I'm nearly ninety, so it was the dark ages. When I was widowed, I did meet a man, and wow, that's when I learnt about real lovemaking. I was over fifty six years at the time. I have met a Buddhist priest, a very understanding and peaceful man, and we have discussed this spiritual side of lovemaking. Once it happens to you, you know it.

So, you've seen a lot of change, then?

Well, yes, I have four children, and only one is still in her first marriage. It seems much easier to get divorced now.

Have you ever discussed your private life, sexuality, etc., with anyone?

Never. I haven't discussed this with anyone before. I have close friends, but we never discuss that. I think I am a product of my growing up. I was born during the Depression, and then there was the war, so I have lived in many different eras. Before I married, I had other boyfriends, but even in nursing, we never discussed sex. In those days, you became a nurse to marry a doctor, and most of my friends did. I didn't.

But you had a chance [laughing] you went out with a medical student.

I know, but he was a Catholic, too. Because I have lived this long, I have experienced so much: raising children, my husband's death at a relatively young age and a love affair. I have an inquiring mind. When I hear of something, I want to hear about it. So, around the sexuality bit, I've read so many books on it. It's a fascinating subject. I am still reading, although because of my eyesight, there are talking books now, and I am still learning. I never knew about masturbation and vibrators. I look at my life now; I have learnt so much and feel somewhat wise now.

It was somewhat embarrassing using certain words when writing this book. For a long time, I used to say "O" for orgasm, but you seem extremely confident using these words.

Oh yes, I can tell them that is no trouble. I'm nearing ninety after all.

So, can we talk about this man in your life?

He wasn't really in my life all the time, but we had the most wonderful relationship. We never lived together, but as far as I was concerned, we were a couple. It was extraordinary for both of us. But it wasn't just lovemaking; I say to my children that sex starts in the kitchen.

You don't mean him doing the washing up, do you?

No, it's more than that. It's being aware of each other. Making love is when he comes into the kitchen and touches you while passing on his way to the fridge. It could be doing the dishes together. That's what having sex as an older woman means. It's not so much as getting into bed and having sex. It's sitting on the couch watching television together, which is intimacy. Sometimes, when my husband was alive, I would tell him I was not wearing undies. I would let him know. It was rather bold of me, really.

Because that's when sex starts, it's not just wham bam, thank you, mam. The Jesuit priests brought up my husband, so it was quite a shock for him.

How do you think women were viewed in society when you were young compared to nowadays?

As I said earlier, I wasn't allowed to use my married name when I went back to work at the hospital. People assumed your husband couldn't support you. He was the head of the family, which was a blow to his pride if you worked. It's like women were the property of men. Now, I think women were viewed as commodities. There weren't many women doctors or lawyers in those days.

That was true in my day, too. In the 1960s, there were only about five women medical students in my year. They were often much cleverer than the men to get a place, but they all became general practitioners; they didn't want to compete with their husbands and become specialists. How many cardiac or neurosurgeons have we lost to that generation?

I had to fight to achieve anything. My father was very much a man of his era, born in 1908. He was the head of the house, and the wife and children did as they were told. My mother never worked outside the home and had never driven a car. I was twenty nine before I got a driving licence myself. I challenged my father sometimes, but only with small things, not big things. I've constantly challenged the status quo. My father wanted me to have a good education, so that is why he sent me to the convent. When I married, I had to promise to "love, honour and obey". My husband took it literally, too; once, when I said I didn't want to have sex, my husband turned to me and said, "But it's my conjugal right." Catholic men believed that in those days, once they were married, they had the right to have sex whenever they wanted. It's sort of in the gospels, too, I think, and even St Paul somewhere said something about it.

That's quite Jewish in a way, isn't it?

Yes, that's because in the Catholic church, once Christ was born, all their ceremonies were still Jewish—they took them on.

So, what are your views on sex, desire and intimacy now?

For us, lovemaking was the two of us coming together as one. It's yin and yang, the penis and the vagina. When we are together as man and woman, we are built like that; it's nature, and when it is right, it's so beautiful. When you come together and have the feeling, you feel like one. I had not experienced that in my marriage. Nick, my lover, brought something new to our relationship, which changed everything. I feel lovemaking is not sex; there must be a spark. When we met, I felt shivers up my whole body. When it happened, we both went to heaven— and not in the Catholic way. Particularly when it happened to us for the first time. Neither of us had experienced it before; it is what we shared. My view is that some people have sex, and some make love. Not every couple has that experience. What I have learned is that men can have an erection quickly, but women take longer to arouse, generally. Lovemaking from the male needs patience and foreplay. That's why women's pleasure has been in the background; if you don't take the time, it is all over for the women, so women are told they are frigid. Men need to be told about this, but my generation was never told that women could enjoy sex. It was all about men. Their job was to make the woman pregnant, according to the Catholics anyway. Neither men nor women ever know enough—they think it will happen naturally, but it won't; lovemaking is a skill. People think it's natural, but it's understanding the difference between men and women, not just our genitals. Sometimes, it is just the chemistry between the two of you. You don't need to be married to have this out of-body experience of togetherness. It rarely happens inside a marriage. It was for both of us. It doesn't have to be a penis. They have other things going for them; it's a burden on men now. In the Catholic church, sex is for procreation. It's all about having as many Catholic children as possible.

Thank you, Maria-Rosa; what you are telling me is worthy of a book all on its own. I could talk to you all day.

I don't think I am old; I've had a good life. On some levels, it's been tragic, but not now.

Dawn [age 77]: There is a Fine Line Between Fury and Desire

I like being married; I like security and protection. I also like being married because, despite my blabbing about women's rights and calling myself a feminist, I have been known to answer a curly question with, "I will have to ask my husband about that."

But sometimes, I don't like him very much, and sometimes, he doesn't like me very much either. Let's be clear: no one apart from the two individuals knows what happens inside a marriage. To the world, we are a perfect couple. People ask me what the secret of a long marriage is. I tell them that I have no idea. Because I don't.

My husband and I have had a few moments when we felt like throwing in the marital towel, but fortunately, not at the same time. We've taken each other up to the brink of divorce and caused so much unpleasantness that our adult children became totally bored by the whole thing. I have disappeared in a huff several times—and so has he. But eventually, one of us comes back.

Sex has been a constant. Despite neither having slept with anyone else—physically, we are completely compatible. Intimacy with him is lovely; he is the only man I have ever desired. Sex was the glue that held us together.

We have even had sex when we were barely speaking. It has put us back on an even keel and made us return to each other—to think again. Sometimes, it wasn't just sex but intimacy and touch that brought us back together. After a huge row, I remember us lying rigidly in our double bed with our backs to each other. I was still furious with him, but I missed him. I waited until he had gone to sleep, then turned over and cuddled up to his back for comfort. He pretended to be still asleep but reached out and put his hand on my encircling arm.

Despite it all, we may hate each other with a passion, but we also love each other with the same passion. We can say the most horrible things to each other and not speak for days. Once he called me an evil bitch, and I was so incredulous and hurt that he thought that about me, so I slapped him around the face so hard that I almost lost my balance. Sometimes, we behave so foolishly that we collapse in laughter at our childishness. Once, I threw a strawberry yoghurt at him, and since he was much younger then, he ducked, and it smashed into the wall behind him. It took us days to get the pigment out of the wallpaper, and the stain sat silently for days, disapproving of our juvenile behaviour.

"That's the last time you will ever speak to me like that, I say, and we sulk around the house, studiously ignoring each other— and then he says the magic words, 'I suppose you wouldn't want a cup of tea, would you?'"

Valerie [age 74]: Vibrators and Viagra

I have never fancied older men, so why would I start now? After my second divorce at the age of 64, I decided that was it as far as sex was concerned. But my neighbour persuaded me to go on a dating site as a joke. It may be alright for the younger generation, but you usually get someone else's cast off when you are older.

After dating older men, internet dating, affairs with married men, and periods of no sex at all, there are two loyal friends that you should never part with your vibrators and Viagra.

Sharon [age 79]: I Learnt More than English Literature at University

I'm an Essex girl, through and through; however, being an Essex girl in the sixties was quite different from being an Essex girl today. The *Oxford English Dictionary* refers to today's Essex girls as, "unintelligent, promiscuous, and materialistic," while Collins adds, "devoid of taste" to the mix.

Neither my school friends nor I were promiscuous or materialistic, and since I went to university much later, I don't consider myself unintelligent. But going to university was when the trouble started. I was captivated and intrigued by the film *Educating Rita* (1983), starring Julie Waters and Michael Caine, because it is almost my story, too.

I married the first man that I had sex with. He was a typical bloodied 20-something-year-old man, and in the beginning, it was undoubtedly about his pleasure. I had no idea about orgasms. I unexpectedly experienced one after a fairly long bout of sex. It took me completely by surprise. I confess I thought I was having an epileptic fit.

My mum had not told me much about sex, just the basics, really; her main thrust was that nice girls didn't, and I would reduce my chances of marriage if people knew I had slept with someone other than my husband.

She slacked off a bit when I became engaged. However, she always put my fiancé and me in separate bedrooms when he came to stay. One night, I had a nightmare and screamed in my sleep. My fiancé ran up the stairs from the room my mum had put him in and lay beside me to calm me down. I later discovered that my mum told my dad not to take a cup of tea to me that morning. As a family, our house was always awash with tea, and my dad always made tea for whoever was in the house in the morning.

After we got married, I was allowed to keep my job as a PE teacher, which was quite unusual as when I was at school, the teachers who got married had to leave. I went to a teachers' training college, and the concept of going to university to obtain a degree was never discussed. University was for two or three exceptional girls in my class.

When Open University became available in the UK, I enrolled almost immediately. I was blown away almost from day one. We read feminist books written by Gloria Steinem, Germaine Greer, Sylvia Plath, Betty Friedan, and feminist theory. I began to see that society prioritised the male point of view and that applied to my marriage. My husband struggled for a while, but my eyes had been opened, and we amicably separated. We had no children, so splitting the assets was simple and uncomplicated. I got the Rolling Stones records, and he got The Beatles.

The Open University required two-week residential courses, and that's when it all began for me. Most of the students went to bars in the evenings. I was missing the intimacy and touch from my marriage, and all of a sudden, I was in a pool of young, intelligent people at the height of their sexuality. They were brilliant to me; I had evenings out, good conversations and sex. As I had only slept with one man up until this point, I went mad. I celebrated my birthday during one of these courses, and my roommate bought me a vibrator as a joke. That was another learning experience. Most of the women had vibrators because they said that very few men had any idea of what they should be doing to pleasure a woman. Straight intercourse rarely led to orgasm, particularly one-night stands.

Later, I had a couple of long-term relationships, but my

heart wasn't in them. To say (the first person I had a long-term relationship with after my divorce was clueless about women's pleasure was an understatement); it was all over in a matter of minutes. I went back to Essex for a while to sort out my mum's stuff and met up with a man I had known from youth club when I was fifteen. He was a widower now, having cared for his wife for many years, who had suffered a brain tumour. I had known them both and knew they had had a loving relationship. We started a sexual relationship, which was very satisfying. Later, he sometimes suffered erectile dysfunction. He decided to go to the hospital to have an implant fitted. I felt all eyes on me when I visited him in hospital. It was OK, although it made our life a bit calculated. But he knew his way around a woman's body; he was a retired doctor, so he hadn't forgotten his anatomy lectures. He knew which buttons to press, to put it crudely. For that reason, too, being medically trained, he knew he was unsuitable to be prescribed Viagra.

His erectile dysfunction didn't bother me. It was the best sex I had ever had, even though I was almost 74. Sex doesn't revolve around erections or orgasms. We are very tactile together. I have a hot tub in the garden, which we sometimes use on a summer evening with a glass of wine each. We have the same sense of humour and see the funny side of most situations, particularly when we have to help each other out of the jacuzzi. What I discovered is that, at the ripe old age of seventy-eight, I am still enjoying sex, but in a completely different way. We have been together a while now, but because of the loving sex life we experienced earlier together, the intimacy we now experience is divine.

Christine [age 67]: The Practicalities of Love Now

My partner is much more romantic than I am. We used to make love nearly every day, but now it depends; it could be once a fortnight or every couple of months.

We both have issues. I have an arthritic knee, and Jeremy has had a hip replacement. I have always preferred the missionary position, as I can almost guarantee an orgasm, but it has been a while since he was on top. Things like positioning the body differently or using cushions to support me can make all the difference. Of course, I have some lubricant in my bedside drawer, and we use a lot of that. I feel a bit embarrassed at the supermarket if it is in my trolley, so I will put a packet of peas on the top.

After I had a hysterectomy, it became a little bit uncomfortable to have penetrative sex. Almost at the same time, Jeremy started having problems getting erect. It all became a bit of an effort. We enjoy cuddling, and if it gets more sexual, then we usually settle for mutual masturbation. My generation feels a bit embarrassed about masturbation, so I would never admit this to my friends. We are embarrassed to say we fake an orgasm, too, but I know all my friends have at some time. Usually, it is because we are not in the mood, and I have done it because Jeremy feels he has failed if I do not. I know Jeremy mourned the loss of his erection for a while, but he has come to terms with it now. Sometimes, he gets a spontaneous erection, and we enjoy that. But even if we do have a physical connection, our intimacy is much deeper now.

Cathy [age 68]: Sharing the Love Around

In the summer of 1974, when books like *The Joy of Sex* and *The Hite Report* hit the bookshelves, everyone seemed to be talking about sex. The 1970s were a time of big changes in society and culture. It felt to me, at least as if we were entering a new world that challenged how we saw love, intimacy and relationships, particularly monogamy. Wife swapping, as it was called then, a once hush-hush topic, was starting to come up in our social circles.

People related stories of "key parties", a party where everyone put their house keys in the centre of a circle and then picked a different one and took their new partner home. I was never going to do that; it sounded far too much like a wife being a possession and being passed around like an old boot. But I was about to experience something, and it came sooner rather than later.

One day, Paul and I were at a party. I saw one of the women from my yoga group lead Paul away upstairs, and then her husband edged towards me. I was nervous but also curious about what might happen. But then I thought, why not follow him? What's fair for Paul is fair for me, too. The experience was a revelation. It wasn't merely about physical pleasure that he gave me. It was about the new experience of sharing yourself—your body, your desires, your vulnerabilities—with someone who wasn't your spouse. It wasn't so much about the sex. It was about intimacy and making a connection with another person. I felt alive.

He smelt and moved differently. His body was completely different from the one I was used to. He had short dark hair and a hairy chest and back. He was not the sort of man I usually fell for. But he was dynamic in bed. I fell in love with him, and he fell in love with me. It's not unusual.

That was a sign to me that this was threatening my marriage. I still loved my husband, but I was addicted to this new man. I got all the usual butterflies from being in love with him, and I behaved like a teenager. Fortunately for my marriage, fate intervened, and he and his wife moved away for work. I was bereft for a while, but after that passed, I was grateful that it ended. I loved my husband; we had children, enjoyed the same things, and had a mortgage.

Looking back decades later, I realise how those experiences shaped my views on intimacy and relationships. They taught me that love is not a finite resource to be stashed away and shared with just one person.

The seventies may be a distant memory now. I am a widow now, but occasionally, I think longingly of how it felt to be loved and adored, but mostly how it felt to become alive at just a simple touch from my lover.

Diana [age 79]: Mum was Ahead of Her Time

As a true Baby Boomer, I was born in the shadow of World War II. The war weighed heavily on our generation and changed so many things.

Yet my mother, born before World War I, was, in a sense, liberated by World War II. When war broke out in 1939, she was married but had no children. She decided she wouldn't wait to be called up and possibly be assigned to work in the land army or a munitions factory. She would determine her destiny, so she joined the Royal Navy. She was a radar plotter. Her sister, who also joined the navy, was responsible for monitoring the shipping off the East coast of England. She told me that being employed again was exciting as she had been obliged to resign from her job as a buyer in a department store when she got married. She had had no choice with that.

I was an only child, so Mum and I spent a lot of time together. She told me about sex at quite an early age. Her friends, too, were quite progressive for the time, and I often overheard them talking about men and intimacy when they came to our house. It had something to do with living in close quarters during the war years.

Many of them had been intimate with their boyfriends, as one never knew if they would survive another day. Hasty marriages before being deployed overseas were very common.

Looking back, I had quite a liberal education. At eleven, I passed an entrance exam and attended an all-girls government grammar school. Most of the teachers had university degrees, and due to the war few men were available, they were unmarried and devoted teachers. They taught us about life and encouraged us to strive for interesting careers. The French teacher went to France during the holidays, and the Latin teacher scoured ancient Greek sites. When they returned, they told us about their adventures.

Whilst some of my friends started to have sex with their boyfriends around [the age of] fifteen, not everyone did. Mostly, we were petrified of getting pregnant. We bombarded the girls who said they had had sex with their boyfriends with questions: "What did it feel like? Did it hurt? Weren't they scared of getting pregnant?"

The girls relied on the boys for contraception. There were no supermarkets with anonymous unmanned cash registers in those days. Buying condoms from the chemist when it might be your aunt behind the counter was unthinkable. So many couples just trusted luck, and the inevitable occurred. I was summoned home one weekend for a family conference. My cousin had become pregnant with her very first boyfriend. My aunt would not hear of them getting married as the boy involved was considered unsuitable, and my cousin duly gave birth to a little girl who was adopted before she had even seen her. My cousin never married or even dated anyone else after that.

I think our parents accepted that we would not be like them and stay virginal until our wedding night. Yet most of my friends married the man with whom they first had sex. So, in a sense, nothing changed.

But we had not had much sexual experience before we met our life's partners, which meant that when that first relationship ended and we started dating again, we were out of touch with how much sex and dating had changed. I believe that the sex education and social conditioning we baby boomers experienced affected how we viewed sex. Sex supposedly started in the sixties with the baby boomers. But in my view, it wasn't until the pill's availability, which came much later, that things changed.

But at least we were taught something about sex, which many of our mother's generation were not.

Sarah [age 82]: Coloured Condoms and My Honeymoon

I was a virgin when I married in 1966, and so was my husband. I was quite apprehensive about the wedding night, although, as a nurse, I knew my anatomy and physiology. But not a lot.

The wedding was at eleven a.m. in the local village church, and my parents erected a marque in their garden. After a traditional breakfast of champagne, chicken sandwiches, vol-au-vents and cakes, we set off for our honeymoon to Bournemouth, a seaside resort on the south coast [of England]eleven. My husband's friends had decorated our car with a "Just Married" sign, with tin cans attached to the bumper. There was much joking and whispering amongst his friends, and I dreaded to think what they had planned. My bridesmaid later told me my mum had stood guard over my suitcase.

After the wedding, we were exhausted and a bit stressed after such a busy day. My dad had driven me into town at about seven in the morning to my hairdresser, Mr David, who had opened early, especially for me. My dad and I were alone in the house before the hired car came to collect us and take us to the church. We had a glass of sherry to calm our nerves. It was just us in the kitchen. Dad, bless him, said, "You look lovely, darling. I am sure there is something I should be saying to you now, some words of advice or something, but I think you will be fine. Your mum and I are very proud of you."

We arrived at the church on time. When we approached, we saw the priest waiting for us outside. My dad turned to me [sitting] in the car's back seat and said, "That's a bit unusual. He should be waiting for us inside at the altar."

The priest told us to drive around the block a few times. There were no mobile phones in those days, so we had no clue what was happening. Eventually, we saw my fiancé's battered old car with him, the best man and his mum inside pull up outside the church. In those days, all the groom's side was obliged to do was organise the flowers—and the cars. He had one job, and he blew it. I struggled down the aisle, furious.

My fiancé had had to travel from his mum's house, about an hour's drive away. He had an old car, and they had a puncture on the way. His mum was in a state because she was late too. She was also worried that her son wasn't wearing a proper wedding tie. It was the height of the sixties, and he had bought himself a flowered tie. When his mum saw him, she said his tie was disrespectful and would look terrible in the photos, so she produced a more suitable silver tie, which caused a further delay.

Despite being nineteen and twenty two years old, respectively, we were shattered by the day's emotions. We finally got to the hotel, brushed the confetti out of our clothes and hair, and found that the best man had slipped some coloured condoms into our luggage. We tentatively started to make love when we first got to bed. I was decked out in a lace negligee that my auntie had bought me. Neither of us had any idea what we were doing. When it came to the condom, we both burst out laughing. We tried a few more times, and then my husband said, "Let's try again in the morning," which we did.

My wedding day is a time capsule of what happened to many young couples in their seventies and eighties. It was a tale of a wedding and social values lost in time.

Abigail [age 82]: Being the Kids of a Vicar Wrecked my Brother's and My Life

Being a Church of England priest, my father was probably the most influential part of my life growing up. In the beginning, my brother and I just had to go to Sunday school a lot more than our friends, but later, the church's teaching was to affect both my and my brother's marriages and how we viewed sex.

Being the children of the local vicar meant we were well versed with phrases such as "living in sin", "unmarried mothers", and "fallen women". Our parents slept in separate beds in the vicarage because they didn't want any more children.

Our parents taught us well that sex before marriage was forbidden. It wasn't just because of religion or that my father was a priest, but it was a universal theme at the time. Mostly, it was because of the fear of pregnancy. It's hard to believe now, but getting pregnant and becoming an unmarried mother in those days was a massive scandal. So, I was blissfully unaware of sex. My mother never mentioned the subject until the night before my wedding, and then only briefly. She said that part of being a wife was to have sexual relations, and it might hurt the first time, but it was part of being married. She could have said, "Lie back and think of England," I was none the wiser of the practicalities and utterly ignorant that it could be enjoyable.

When I was still at school, my brother severely challenged my father's faith and religious teachings and caused a rift in the family from which we never recovered. One weekend, he came down to the vicarage with his girlfriend. My mother put them in separate bedrooms. After Matins on Sunday, my brother and his girlfriend said they had something to tell us. We assembled in the sitting room, unsure what was coming up. My brother announced his girlfriend was pregnant and asked my dad if he would marry them. I was quite excited to become an auntie and assumed they would marry a bit earlier than they were planning. All would be well, but then my dad spoke. He replied that he would have been able to marry them if they hadn't told him she was pregnant but now he knew that she was, he couldn't. My father said the church teaching was quite specific; he could not in all conscience marry a couple who had lived in sin. The sad ending to this story is my brother and his girlfriend left for London the next day and married in a registry office; none of us were invited or attended. When their child arrived, my father wouldn't even christen his granddaughter. My brother and his wife left for Canada shortly after, and I didn't see him again for many years.

Rachel [age 74]: A Jewish Perspective

Where do I begin?

My journey began in an old post-war army ambulance at the age of two days, as my mother and I bounced across an Egyptian desert—not sand but very uneven centuries worn wadi rocks. A young British army driver had been assigned to our journey in the heat of the day and through unchartered territory. At the time, my young British parents were stationed at a Royal Air Force base in Suez. As the story goes, my mother had not made it to the RAF base hospital for my delivery. The nearest choice had been a basic army facility that, due to stringent British services protocol, needed to transport us both to our British RAF base and compound within days of my birth, as we were not their responsibility or personnel.

I first became a wife at the very young age of twenty one. It was early in the 1970s. Motown and Merseyside music stirred my soul. Leonard Cohen sang pure poetry and the truth of love and life. Drugs, sex and rock 'n' roll liberated and began to free a generation breaking at the seams to be different, heard and rebellious.

The 1980s also saw a major shift towards the emergence of

a global gay culture. [My] marriage lasted a difficult eighteen years. Shrouded in the secrecy of my husband's struggle with his hidden sexuality and dalliances, I peddled on through most of the years trying to survive the long silences, his untold anger, lack of communication, true love and intimacy, and, of course, my own sense of loss, betrayal and displacement.

I left the marriage with only a small amount of cash in my purse. I had borrowed money for a lease on a small bedroom flat and promised my two sons, who were fifteen years old and nine, that I would return to collect them. A single mother of two in my late thirties, I struggled with no support. My ex-husband, a successful lawyer by then, and still in a time where the codes and morals of society placed a heavy stigma upon homosexuality, caused us to batten down our hatches, and we began to live as a family of silence.

I became a wife for the second time at the age of 46 years. By then, I had been drawn into what seemed to outside eyes a deeply spiritual existence of order, conformity, predictability, and ancient laws that had stood the test of time. They would guide my very existence, sense of community, thinking and understanding of self! Beyond the fringes of the prayer shawl or tallit that each married man wore during daily morning prayers, their wives appeared radiant, united and secure. Protected! I was the third wife of my second husband—a man with a sense of charm and a roving eye for female attention. Raised in an age-old religion where ancient laws to this day still directed every aspect of life, his days were seemingly filled with unbending instructions, observance, directives, statute, regulations and rules. His daily morning prayers, said just as the sun was rising and as he sat almost protected under his tallit, in peace and away from my presence, contained a particular section in which he would fervently thank God for not making him a woman.

Modesty, or being tzniut, was the foundation of the ancient laws and their values. Modesty not only meant the concept of dress but also involved behaviour, simplicity and reserve. A modest woman, a very specific quality, makes an ideal 'mate'. Marriage was believed to be a contact between a man and a woman in which God was involved. A marriage can end with the process of a divorce document or get, given by the man to his wife, drawn up and issued by an all-male court or bet din, a bench of what is considered learned men who spend hours, days, months and years of their lives studying the ancient laws. On the day of my get, I was unaware that my then-husband had arranged the final ending of our 20-year-old marriage, to be now able to enjoy a new relationship with someone almost thirty years his junior. The ridding of me would ensure he could rest beside her with an easy mind by observing the necessary rules of divorce and acting according to the law. I asked to receive my marriage contract, or ketubah, drawn up and signed on my wedding day to keep me provided for, happy and protected; it was now folded and cut in several places to be dropped into my cupped hands. This was to allow all in the room to witness my understanding of the finality and end of the marriage.

Throughout the 20 years of this marriage, the roots of doubt and endless struggle to maintain my sense of self-worth, true value, independence, happiness, and fulfilment, particularly sexual, spread through every inch of my life. I had learnt to walk in his shadow. I was there to ensure his happiness, fulfilment, and desire. I don't remember any moment of his being concerned or even caring enough to explore the realms of my needs or sexuality. Any barriers set up within the laws that pertain to women, their security, happiness and true value have been seemingly set up and maintained to this day under the guise of protection. I had not been up on a pedestal but in a cage. The image of the desolate desert trek of my childhood and my absent father has always been a reference point in my mind of the often never-questioned expectations of women—their unfulfilled needs and automatic compliance. The developing years of my childhood and early memories of a life of military discipline, hierarchy, codes and rules governed my relationships. They determined the pathways and the quality of my life.

Jenny [age 72]: I Had the Best Sex of my Life at 42. It Obviously Wasn't With My Husband

Sometimes, the greatest relationships are the ones you never expect to be in. I got swept off my feet and disrupted every moral code I believed in. I was quite ignorant of sex before I got married in 1978. All the sex, drugs and rock 'n' roll of the seventies had passed me by.

I trained as a primary school teacher, and only a few men were in my college. There was one—and I married him. He later became a headmaster at a government school while I devoted myself to bringing up our two daughters. My family were church-going

Presbyterians, so I was a virgin when I married.

When my children were relatively young, my husband became involved in a project for underprivileged children and went overseas for six weeks to work as a volunteer. Whilst he was away, I often saw an old friend who had children at the same school as my children. His wife was away quite a lot, visiting her ageing parents. So, we were both alone, and he helped me out with my kids, taking them swimming and things like that. One day after he had taken us all to the zoo, it was quite late, so he stayed over in the spare room, but not for long.

It was the most beautiful six weeks of my life. I would say that those first few weeks of the affair were a heady mix of bliss and pain, which is what one must expect from an extramarital affair. My lover had had several relationships at university, so he knew what he was doing. I experienced oral sex for the first and only time in my life. I had no idea that people did this; it was bliss, all the attention on me. It felt so natural that I did the same to him—because I wanted to! I decided not to tell my husband because what was the point? It would only cause more heartache. Several months later, my husband saw photos of us in a group photo at a wedding and asked me about him. Body language doesn't lie. We looked very happy together, rightly so, as we were ridiculously in love.

What hurts the most is that we never really said goodbye. It just sort of ended. But when it's over, you will be sad for a while, and then eventually, you stop giving a fuck, and it's the best feeling ever. But there is no easy solution to forgetting someone. It's just something you must endure until you don't anymore. I drift between celebrating and regretting my actions, but ultimately, I would firmly come down on the side of the celebration: a guilty secret, perhaps, but one I treasure.

Alice [age 73]: I have Been Married Fifty Years, Ten Were a Bit Shit, But Mostly, it Was Good

I think Michelle Obama said something quite similar but it sums up my and many of my friend's marriages.

Whilst still officially married, we have long stopped being joined at the hip. Often, it's because one or another in the marriage has developed some disability or has just lost interest. There have been many ups and downs in a long time together, and my husband and I have had our fair share. I have discussed this with many of my friends and goddaughter, who have shown remarkable insight.

She believes, and I think she is on the money, that men turn into grumpy old men around sixty. Not all, of course; some men adapt very well to retirement, taking on new hobbies, sometimes newer younger partners, and enjoying what they have left. It's all to do with feeling respected and loved. A lot of men, particularly those born after 1945, define themselves by their jobs. If they were heads of departments, CEOs, hot shot lawyers or specialist surgeons, commanding respect, then it's a big blow when they retire.

One friend of mine was the CEO of a large Australian organisation and described it thus: "One day, you are driven to the airport in a fancy BMW, ushered into first class for a comfortable flight and then put up in a five-star hotel. The day after, when you have retired and taking a family holiday, it all changes. You drive yourself to the airport in a car that still smells of dog hair, find a parking space, struggle through security and find yourself in the back of the aircraft with the rest of the world. Welcome to Civvy Street, Sir—no wonder you are grumpy."

Georgia [age 82]: Online Dating

I was alone for the first time and missed my partner. We had been together for sixty years. All our friends were couples. I did not belong to a club where I could meet other people, including men, so I thought the obvious place to look for a companion was online. It seemed quite logical.

I enrolled on a site and was overwhelmed by the responses, many from incredibly young men. By young, I mean forty–fifty-year-olds. I knew nothing about how dating apps worked, but lucky me, one was a decent man. However, it did not work out for many reasons, and I left the site soon afterwards. I was watching TV once and heard a woman in an audience discussing older dating say,

"There are lovely people out there, but they are not on dating apps."

I agree with her. I met one man who had issues that alarmed me a bit. So, I advise that in some situations, you may have to block someone who persists in making contact. Ensure you understand how your phone works and the guidelines for safely using the internet; there are rules and guidelines. I would say that knowing them before you step into the big online world is essential. However, the dating experience made me think about my needs and how to describe what I was looking for. It was wanting someone to share a walk, go to a play, or have a meal with, which seems straightforward.

Susan [age 72]: My Marriage Went Down When His Willy Didn't Go Up

I am in my sixties and grew up in Australia, so the sexual revolution came a bit later for us than in the UK.

I had a conservative upbringing, and my family didn't discuss sex at home. I had a few previous relationships before marrying, but nothing serious. My husband was my first boyfriend. I don't have much to compare it with, as although I had an older sister, I was ignorant about what other people did sexually. I would say that we had a relatively everyday life until my husband became ill. Then everything changed.

My husband had been experiencing difficulties with having an erection; in fact, that was what drove him to the doctor in the first place. He became very depressed when his body didn't cooperate with his desires, and there was unquestionable tension between us. After the prostate cancer surgery, it was a dark time for both of us.

Initially, we were so relieved that he was still alive, although the surgeon advised us that there might be some sexual dysfunction, which we both agreed was a horrible word. The doctors advised us that some medications and devices were available to us. We talked about them, but they weren't really for us. The emphasis was on the mechanics of sex.

My husband did try Viagra. We were warned that as he was borderline hypertensive, there could be problems. With all his other medical issues, we thought he had enough on his plate without complicating things, so he didn't take it. We never argued about the situation as we both felt anxious about discussing sex. But we grew distant as he thought I was coming on to him whenever I tried to cuddle him. So, in the end, we became even more detached. We still shared a bed, but it was as if we were brother and sister. I still feel sexual urges and would love to have some form of physical intimacy, even if it wasn't like before. We still love each other, but now it is more like we are housemates.

Mary [age 65]: A Dating Agency in The 1980s

I was a model in the sixties; it wasn't really anything I had planned. I was spotted when I had a Saturday job at the local hairdressers in my town. I wasn't on the front page of Vogue or anything like that, but I made a good living.

Some of my friends started sexual relationships, but in those days, before the pill, we were always scared to get pregnant, so we didn't have the wild sex life that everyone imagined. But we used condoms, and I had quite a few serious boyfriends. Perhaps it was the circle I moved in, but the men knew about women's pleasure—possibly from the sex manuals that had started drifting into the bookshops.

I married a photographer at a registry office, not in a white dress, but in navy blue, which was the fashion at the time. Celebrities rarely play by the rules. In London in the 1960s, it was about rebellion against what our parents had done; nothing was conventional about famous brides and grooms then. Linda McCartney (wife of Beatle Paul), Audrey Hepburn, and Liz Taylor all married in miniskirts. In those days, we didn't wear huge white dresses; there was an ongoing joke that you wouldn't get married in white if you weren't entitled to. My husband and I had a wonderful few years, but I wanted to settle down, and he was hell-bent on making his mark as a society photographer. We divorced, and both went our separate ways.

Shortly after, I met a man who ticked all the boxes for solidarity and security, and we had two children. Unfortunately, our happiness was short-lived as he died quite suddenly from a brain tumour. Brain disease was a death sentence in those days.

I returned to work as a model, which suited me well as I could pick and choose what hours I would work. I joined a modelling agency and settled into photographic work, which was quite dull, but it paid the bills. I did mostly photographic work with a bit of catwalk thrown in, but photographic modelling was where the money was in those days. Catalogue shopping was quite the thing during this time, as women could browse what they would buy in the privacy of their own homes. I also appeared in a lot of knitting patterns.

But I was lonely, so one of my friends encouraged me to join a dating agency. Since this wasn't widespread in those days like today, I didn't tell many people. I enrolled in a relatively exclusive and expensive agency in London, hoping perhaps I would meet someone compatible. I could afford it because I had earned reasonable money modelling.

I met Nigel almost in the first match. He had been divorced and had a couple of children. We went out for dinner several times to some excellent restaurants, and I felt sufficiently confident that I could spend a weekend with him in his cottage. He gave me a spare room very gallantly; he was old school, and I liked that. Eventually, one thing led to another, and we slept together.

The sex was a bit uninspiring to begin with, probably because he had been brought up very strictly and went to a boy's school. A friend gave us a box of chocolates that featured chocolate figures in various positions, probably inspired by the Kama Sutra. I set about educating him about sex; at first, he was a bit shocked, but eventually, we settled into a perfect sex life.

The younger generation who rely on internet dating might have a different experience today.

Heather [age 77]: My Husband's Affair Changed Everything

I was smitten when I first saw my [future] husband in my first year of university. He wasn't conventionally handsome, but he had an easy, relaxed charm that was utterly beguiling. He was funny as well as self-effacing, everything I was not.

I had been to a conventional all-girls school and was somewhat uncomfortable with boys, even though I had two brothers. I was shy with boys, and although I was relatively presentable looks-wise, I wasn't a classic beauty. Like all my siblings, I was clever, so I tended to concentrate on that, although I knew instinctively at the time that boys preferred pretty girls with big breasts.

My husband had had a few girlfriends, which added to his charm because he was very confident around women. Women were in the minority in my year, so I concentrated on doing well. I tried to play it down, and when we married, I decided that there could only be one highflyer in the family, so I took a much less important job than his.

Looking back at the photos of our early years together, I am looking at him, completely besotted. I had had one boyfriend before him, so I had some experience, but that was it. It was tough in the sixties to find private time to have sex. Later generations would find it hard to believe, but hotels were not keen to have unmarried couples stay with them, and you had to buy a cheap ring from Woolworths and say you were married. But we were students and couldn't afford to stay in hotels.

So, to get around this, we often spent our weekends in the countryside, taking a tent with us. Even though we were engaged then, my mother was visibly distressed when I told her I was camping on the weekends with my fiancé. So we went to enormous trouble, took two small tents, duly photographed them, and sent them to my parents. I am sure my parents were not convinced, but I was conforming to society's rules then.

When we got married, my husband said he didn't like the idea of condoms anymore, so I dutifully went to the doctor, who inserted a Copper-7 intrauterine device (IUD). I took some Valium before the consultation to relax and calm my nerves. Despite this, it was still very unpleasant, and I remember feeling resentful that I had to undergo that painful procedure just because he didn't like condoms. Although the IUD successfully prevented pregnancy, it caused me some distress. I had bleeding and discomfort. In 1987, there was a class action in Australia against the makers of the intrauterine device, claiming it caused pelvic inflammatory disease. Although I adored my husband, I wouldn't say I enjoyed sex that much. It was hard for me to have an orgasm, but eventually, I found that if I was on top, I could achieve it. I knew it was important for my marriage to succeed and that my husband should be happy sexually.

But he wasn't—obviously—because he had an affair. I was devastated when he confessed to me, and I went into a deep depression which lasted well over six months.

He promised he had broken up with his lover, and I believe he did, although I kept him on a very tight leash after that. I knew the woman; she was a close friend, and I felt betrayed. Looking back at the reasons he had an affair, I think we were both to blame. Sex wasn't that important to me, although I did make a concerted effort to be available to him. If either of us was going to be away, I ensured we had sex before either of us left. My best friend jokingly said, 'Never send your partner off with a loaded gun.' My husband was much more romantic than me, and I think he wanted to be in love, which we were, but not in the way he wanted. Yes, I think we had sex, but we did not make love.

Pauline [age 76]: Sex with Simon Was like a Bush Turkey Scrabbling Around in a Compost Heap

Am I the only one grateful that I no longer need or want to have a physical relationship with a man? Most of my friends, too, have given up on sex, certainly the married ones; if they are having sex at all, it is not with each other. It's not just the sex either; I don't want to share my house with a man.

I am a widow. My husband left me well-provided, and I bought a lovely little apartment near the beach. A Greek coffee shop was situated about 6 metres from my apartment, and I enjoyed my early morning cup of tea with the seagulls and the occasional banter with my neighbours. What was there not to like?

I had a very happy marriage for forty years, but when my husband died, friends and my kids seemed hell-bent on finding me a new man. I missed the comfort of a warm body next to mine, which I had had for so long. I particularly missed the intimacy of being with someone. I did try, but the men that I was introduced to all wanted a sexual relationship very early on.

I met Simon, who said he had been divorced from his wife. He wasn't. I realised it was a big mistake the day he moved in. One day,

I came home from shopping to find a vast removal truck parked in my allocated space. I couldn't believe what he unloaded. Heavy Chinese rosewood furniture and black scuffed leather couches swamped my little bijou apartment with its white linen sofas, carefully chosen artwork, pale blue silk cushions and an Afghan carpet I had bought in a market when backpacking in my youth. Simon was not very tidy either and he had far too much stuff. He had been a serious tennis player, his son was quite famous, and he had racquets, balls and tons of tennis memorabilia from Wimbledon. He also left plates unwashed in the sink overnight and left the toilet seat up.

After all, men, if they are in their sixties or seventies and have been married, have as much stuff as you have. And then there were his Bee Gee records. I hate the Bee Gees.

The sex was very much on his terms, not the loving sex I had enjoyed with my husband. I don't think he could find the clitoris to save his life. A typical male response was when he said that he hadn't had any complaints before. The last straw was when we had some friends for supper, and he said, 'Let me show you around our apartment and explain what we have done.' All he had done was move in—horrible furniture and all. It was time to show him out.

Lorna [age 81]: My First Husband Was Sexually Violent, But it Wasn't Called Rape Then

Growing up, my only social life was in the village tennis club. It was not very inspiring, but that was all there was. So, I was very excited when my best friend's brother arrived home, from where he was training to be a naval officer. He didn't know many girls, so he invited me to his graduation ball. I was awestruck by the formal dining with elaborate silver on the tables, being served by uniformed flunkeys and dancing with dashing men in their dress uniforms.

My parents were delighted when we got engaged. When we married, Dan wore his naval uniform, and we walked out of the church under the crossed swords of his fellow shipmates. It was a whirlwind of romance, and all my dreams had come true.

I initially adored my handsome sailor husband and took to the social life of being part of a community. I had status and ready-made friends.

Dan spent much time with his fellow officers from the ship

and once declined my suggestion of a holiday away so that he could be with them at some naval functions. It should have been a red flag, but I was very innocent in those days. He explained that it was traditional and that he would play ridiculous games and get drunk.

I formed close relationships with the other wives. When the ship was due back after being away, the other wives joked about preparing themselves for the expected sexual marathon on their husband's return. One even changed her contraceptive pill cycle, with the help of the naval doctor, so that she was not having her period when her husband returned for the few days before they set sail again. The sexual marathon never occurred for Dan and me; on one occasion, we didn't have sex, even when he had been away for three months.

For most of our marriage, sex was almost non-existent. Whenever we did have sex, it was always about him. To say he was clueless about women's pleasure was an understatement; it was all over in a matter of minutes. There was never any foreplay or tenderness. He lay on top of me; there was a bit of thrusting, and then he rolled off and started snoring. But even that stopped. I was worried that he didn't find me attractive anymore. One night, after we were lying in bed, I decided to bite the bullet and asked him if there was anything wrong and why he didn't want to have sex with me.

He turned to me and said, 'So you want sex, do you?' Without saying anything, he launched himself upon me quite violently. I didn't think it was rape then, as we were married, but now I do. There was blood on the sheets in the morning, and we never had sex or discussed it again. Forty years later, on reflection, I suspect that he may have been bisexual or gay, but such was my ignorance. I didn't have a clue what that meant. Growing up, I never knew about such things.

My marriage was not happy, but it wasn't unhappy either, and since my parents were still alive, who would have been upset by divorce, we stayed together. My husband died aged 45 from a heart attack. I was now a widow, relatively young and still presentable —and how things changed. Men came out of the woodwork and told me they had always found me attractive. I even had an affair with a married man, which I later learned was very common with newly widowed women. It's called widow's fire, I believe.

Considering that statistically, the chance of finding a new partner at my age is the same as being shot by a terrorist, I was lucky enough to meet my last partner. He knew all about my life with Dan and our problems. We moved in together after a few years, and I am still happily living with him. The longing for affection, the longing for touch and the warmth of another body next to mine is lovely. We cuddle up most nights, and while we sometimes have sex, it's mostly falling asleep in each other's arms. It is a great comfort that someone cares about me, as sexist as it sounds. I belong to someone.

Gwen [age 86]: Late-Life Blooming

I didn't know any women in their 1980s who enjoyed a new romance, so I wasn't expecting it to happen to me. Somehow, I seem to have accepted that I am in what's probably the last stage of my life, though I'd never thought much about it. And besides, it just isn't what we've always believed about what it is to be an older woman.

Octogenarians and romance don't appear in the media— magazines, broadsheets, or online platforms. It's not an image people know about, but I began to think about it once I was plunged into solo living for the first time.

I'm from the era of Saturday night dinner parties and Sunday picnics. So, in my new single life, I joined a local organisation and am gradually finding it more accessible to front up, be prepared not to know anyone there, and begin introducing myself. I am surprised because that part is more accessible than when I was young. I am also reminded of other significant changes in socialising since I was young. Women can and do initiate meetings. It's all-new, but somehow, it's very familiar. And when I meet someone who suggests we have coffee, I am always interested in trying it.

I have met several men whose company I enjoy, and we meet alone or with others to spend an evening with them. This was never how life was when I was young. But it is now, and I'm learning to live differently and be with people of different ages.

I'm surprised by my enjoyment of being courted. I probably believed what everyone else does about older women: that they are past love and desire. It's not true!

Alexander [age 77]: The Casseroles From Women Started Arriving Shortly After My Wife's Death

I never knew that my life would change so dramatically until my wife died. Whilst she was ill, it was a gruelling time, and I nursed her at home for the last two years. Eventually, I sold the big family home and moved into a small modern house in the same village.

Then, the casseroles began arriving! One day, a friend visiting from overseas went to my fridge to get some milk for a cup of tea. 'What are all these pots in your fridge, Alex?' I sheepishly replied that they just kept arriving. They were from my late wife's, mostly divorced and widowed friends. I didn't realise what was happening until I visited my son in the US, and my daughter-inlaw spelt it out.

I was quietly sitting in the garden getting over jet lag in the US when an old friend of my wife's rang my son. She said she was passing through and asked if she could call around for a coffee. The 'passing through' lasted two weeks, but I remained oblivious until my daughter-in-law told me, 'Dad, she's got the hots for you.' I had never been hot in my entire life!

It was bizarre to be pursued and desired at last. I have always been a long-distance runner, so I was fit and reasonably off. A good pension fund is what women want these days! But I took the easy route and settled into a relationship with a mutual friend. We never pretended it was a grand love affair. After my wife died, I wasn't so much looking for love as companionship. Anything to heal the gap in my life. It was practical, too; my wife did everything in the house. I didn't even know how the washing machine worked. I didn't know a lot about sex, either.

Even though it was in the early 1960s, my wife and I didn't have sex until we were married. It was probably unusual because I knew most of my friends of the same age were having noisy sex with their girlfriends. After all, I had lived in a hall of residence, and the walls between our rooms were thin.

So, on our wedding night, it was our first time together. I then realised what I was missing, and I just wanted sex all the time. But my wife was not so keen—we did have two children, so it must have happened now and again. I didn't talk to anyone about this because men certainly didn't talk about the lack of sex—if they said anything, it was about football or cars.

If that all sounds miserable, it wasn't all bad. I did fall hopelessly in love out of the blue with one of my wife's school friends. I drove her home from a function, and as she sat in the seat next to me, I felt an almost unbearable longing and desire for her. She was palpably a woman, and I wanted her. It was a coup de foudre, as the French say. I still don't know what happened, but it was as if Cupid's arrow had struck me. I would be with her now if she hadn't been married.

We hadn't slept together, but for the first time, I longed to be with her all the time. I even texted her, 'I wish I were in bed with you right now,' which is not what I thought 74-year-old grandfathers would ever send to a 75-year-old grandma.

My daughter, a psychologist, picked it up immediately. She said it would have caused a massive scandal for our two families. For God's sake, we were in our seventies! When can we stop doing what other people tell us?

My daughter told me to cut off all contact with her, which I did. To my shame, I ghosted her. I must have caused unbelievable suffering by simply not having the courage to tell her face-to-face. I bolted. I even cut off contact with our mutual friends, which raised many questions and hurt. We were part of an extended family and usually met at least every couple of months. But now? I have never seen her again.

Mark [age 77]: Sex Has Ruled My Life

They say that humans face seven significant decisions in life, and sex made all those decisions for me. I have probably slept with about 20 women, some of whom I have loved and some with whom I have had recreational sex. I was merely eighteen when I became a father for the first time. I got my first girlfriend pregnant. Society was such in the 1960s that I had to get married. I knew I wasn't in love with her, but we did the right thing and married.

My wife was a devoted Catholic, so the rhythm method of contraception, so beloved by the Pope at the time, was her birth control of choice. Does it work? Well, we went on to have three more children. So, no. By the time of the last pregnancy, I knew our marriage was in its death-rattle phase. I began to look elsewhere.

The sex opportunities were there. One night, I was staying with a school friend and his partner, and when I got up to go to the bathroom, I heard noises coming from their bedroom. Their door was open, and as I passed, my friend leaned on his elbow and said, "Care to join us?" It was the eighties, and sex was freely available. It was quite the thing amongst my friends at the time, and sometimes, it was called wife swapping, which indicates the time it was. It has a new name now: polyamorous, I think.

Sex made me make so many mistakes, but eventually, I fell in love for the first time. She became pregnant, too, but it was now the nineties, and she had an abortion without telling me. One night, I confessed all to my heartbroken wife; she was devastated. Strangely, being a Catholic, she was more upset by the abortion than anything else. It was a very dark time. My marriage ended, my girlfriend left me, and I often thought of the baby that might have been. I was in love with my girlfriend, and even to this day, I think of her and wish things had turned out better. But it was not to be. I lost my job, my wife divorced me and took me to the cleaners. I had no home and no money.

During this time, I had little contact with my kids as they made it clear that they were disgusted with me and blamed me for my wife's misery. They all got married in the next few years, but I was not involved in the usual way that fathers are in their children's weddings. I could not walk my daughter down the aisle or appear in any photographs. My son was particularly angry with me, and when it became his time to get married, he didn't even invite me to his wedding but I knew the date and the church, so I snuck into the back of the church as he and his new wife left and pushed some money into his pocket.

My hormones still drove me, and I had several unusual episodes during the next few years. I now had a good job and lived alone in a major city. I was quite the novelty in some circles and had liaisons with some minor celebrities and once a high ranking political figure. In idle moments, I look at their Wikipedia profiles. There is no mention of me, naturally.

Eventually, I met another woman at work and married for the second time. She was a career woman with no children, and as I didn't want any more kids, she was ideal. For many years, we were happy, and then my wife just went off sex. She was going through menopause, but that shouldn't have had the effect it did but being a male, I blamed it. Sex had never been a big part of our lives and she found sex uncomfortable. I felt we could still enjoy intimacy and comfort that didn't require penetrative sex, but she wouldn't let me anywhere near her. It's sad because I wasn't bothered if we didn't have full sex, as I like oral sex. I particularly like watching women orgasm. I must be one of the few men who don't enjoy fellatio. It's okay. It just isn't vital. I often joke with friends my age about the three stages of life for older men: gardening, golf, and grandchildren. I don't do any of those. Perhaps they envy me, and perhaps, at times, I envy them.

XVI

References

I: Introduction

Ageing and Health Report, World Health Organisation. (1 Oct 2025). https://www.who.int/news-room/fact-sheets/detail/ageing-and-health.

World Population Ageing 2023 Report, United Nations. (2023). https://www.un.org/development/desa/pd/sites/www.un.org.development.desa.pd/files/undesa_pd_2024_wpa2023-report.pdf.

Jane Fonda, *Book Club* (2018) press interviews.

Chapter II: What Do Older Women Really Want?

Roger Angell, quoted reflections on ageing and love.

Jane Fonda, *Book Club* (2018) press interviews.

General Population Studies. (2000s–2020s). Australian and UK ageing sexuality surveys.

Chapter III: Still Sexy After All These Years

Kathy Lette, essays and columns on ageing and sexuality.

Emma Thompson, *Good Luck to You, Leo Grande* (2022).

Liz Jones, *Daily Mail* columns on dating, beauty, and ageing.

Chapter IV: Growing Up in the Fifties and Sixties

Beckman.N., *Secular Trends in Self-Reported Sexual Activity*, BMJ 2008;337:a279

UK Department of Education archives on sex education, 1950s–1960s

Campbell, P., Sex education books for young adults, 1892–1979.

The landmark Lady Chatterley's Lover obscenity trial in the UK, *Regina v. Penguin Books Ltd.*, (1961 Crim LR 176)

D. H. Lawrence, *Lady Chatterley's Lover*, 1928

Chapter V: God, Sex, and What Will the Neighbours Say

Seneca, philosophical writings on religion and power.

Encyclical Letter Humanae Vitae of the Supreme Pontiff, Paul VI, The Holy See, 1968

Marc A, Shampo, Phd, and Robert A. Kyle, MD, *"John Rock: Pioneer in the Development of Oral Contraceptives"*, Mayo Clin Press, July 2004, https://www.mayoclinicproceedings.org/article/S0025-6196(11)62148-4/fulltext

Orthodox Jewish prayer texts and feminist theological critiques.

Indonesian Criminal Code revisions (2022).

Chapter VI: Secret Women's Business

Germaine Greer, *The Female Eunuch* (1970).

O'Connell, Helen E., Kalavampara V. Sanjeevan, & John M. Hutson. *Anatomy of the Clitoris*. The Journal of Urology 174 (2005): 1189–95.

Chivers, M. L., & Brotto, L. A. (2017). *Controversies of women's sexual arousal and desire*. European Psychologist, 22(1), 5–26. https://doi.org/10.1027/1016-9040/a000274

Chivers ML, Rieger G, Latty E, Bailey JM. *A sex difference in the specificity of sexual arousal*. Psychol Sci. 2004 Nov;15(11):736-44. doi: 10.1111/j.0956-7976.2004.00750.x. PMID: 15482445.

Tiefer, L., Hall, M., & Tavris, C. (2002). *Beyond Dysfunction: A New View of Women's Sexual Problems*. Journal of Sex & Marital Therapy, 28(sup1), 225–232. https://doi.org/10.1080/00926230252851357

Perel. E. *Mating in Captivity.* (2006).

Edward Laumann, *Sexual Dysfunction in the United States.* JAMA (1999).

Moynihan, Ray. *The making of a disease: female sexual dysfunction.* (2003 Jan 04). BMJ 2003;326:45

Chapter VII: Secret Men's Business

Barry McCarthy, sex therapy research.

John Lloyd: "People on the tennis circuit have since spoken to me about prostate cancer". Prostate Cancer UK. (2018). https://prostatecanceruk.org/about-us/news-and-views/2018/6/john-lloyd#

Henry Marsh. *And Finally* (2017).

Kristie L. Kahl, *Testosterone levels show steady decrease among young US men,* Urology Times Journal - Yale School of Medicine. (2020

Jul 3). Vol 48 No 7.

Lokeshwar SD, Patel P, Fantus RJ, Halpern J, Chang C, Kargi AY, Ramasamy R. *Decline in Serum Testosterone Levels Among Adolescent and Young Adult Men in the USA.* Eur Urol Focus. 2021 Jul;7(4):886-889. doi: 10.1016/j.euf.2020.02.006. Epub 2020 Feb 18. PMID: 32081788.

Dr Chris Church is a nom de plume: GP interviews and clinical experience.

Spritz, Aaron. MD. *The Penis Book.* Rodale. 2018

Chapter VIII: Mind the Gap

Frederick DA, John HKS, Garcia JR, Lloyd EA. *Differences in Orgasm Frequency Among Gay, Lesbian, Bisexual, and Heterosexual Men and Women in a U.S. National Sample.* Arch Sex Behav. 2018 Jan;47(1):273-288. doi: 10.1007/s10508-017-0939-z. Epub 2017 Feb 17. PMID: 28213723.

Wetzel. G.M. Cultice R.A. Sanche. D.T. *Orgasm Frequency Predicts Desire and Expectation for Orgasm: Assessing the Orgasm Gap within Mixed-Sex Couples.* Sex Roles. (2022). 86:456–470

Perel. E. *Mating in Captivity.* (2006).

Chapter IX: Mission Possible: Closing the Gap

Wednesday Martin, *Untrue* (2018).

The Little Death (2014) Australian film.

Emma Thompson, *Good Luck to You, Leo Grande* (2022).

Bianca P. Acevedo, Arthur Aron, Helen E. Fisher, and Lucy L. Brown, *Neural correlates of long-term intense romantic love*. (2011). https://www.helenfisher.com/downloads/articles/Acevedo-et-alLong-term.pdf

Joan Collins interviews on marriage and mystery.

Prue Leith interviews on living apart together.

Chapter X: Love, Lust and Lies

Book of Common Prayer. (1549).

Mason Cooley (1927-2002) was an American aphorist and professor of philosophy.

Glass. S. *Not Just Friends.* (2003).

Ashley Madison surveys (self-reported data).

Selterman. D. *Johns Hopkins University* research. https://www.dylanselterman.com/

Perel. E. *Mating in Captivity.* (2006).

Perel. E. *The secret to desire in a long-term relationship.* TED Talk. (2013).

Perel. E. *Rethinking infidelity ... a talk for anyone who has ever loved.* TED Talk. (2015).

Shere Hite, *The Hite Report.* (1976).

Miriam Margolyes, Three Men and One OUTRAGEOUS Story. Graham Norton Show. (2025).

Chapter XI: Divorce, Death and Dating

Andrews. J. Advancing the Science and Practice of Nursing Practical advice based on evidence. A collection of articles by Fellows of the Royal College of Nursing (UK) to celebrate the International Year of the Nurse and the Midwife 2020. p78. *When people most need it: producing a guide on dementia by June Andrews (FRCN 2014*

Australian Institute of Health and Welfare, dementia statistics.

Prue Leith, interviews on later-life love.

Chapter XII: Navigating Love and Loneliness

Sally Phillips, public commentary on women and pleasure.

Joan Baez, song lyrics and interviews.

Joan Rivers, interviews and stand-up commentary on ageing.

SBS Insight program discussions on intimacy and sex work.

Bowen. N. *Rhonda and Ketut as the faces of female sex tourism.* (2013). https://www.abc.net.au/news/2013-01-22/bowen---ketut/4476716

Gallop. C. TED Talk on porn and sexuality. *Make love, not porn.* (2009). https://www.ted.com/talks/cindy_gallop_make_love_not_porn

Chapter XIII: Love and Intimacy in Aged Care

Dr Daniel Kaplan, geriatric psychiatry research.

Uniting Care NSW aged-care policy statements.

Alison Rahn, Tiffany Jones, Carry Bennett and Amy Lykins, Conflicting Agendas: The Politics of Sex in Aged Care, 2016, https://classic.austlii.edu.au/au/journals/ElderLawRw/2016/4.pdf.

Australian Department of Health, STI statistics over age 65.

Netflix TV Series Grace and Frankie (2015).

Dorking. M.C. *Condoms launched at garden centres after rise in STIs in over 65s*. Yahoo Life, (2022). https://uk.style.yahoo.com/ condoms-launched-garden-centres-rise-st-is-over-65s-104738540. html.

www.ingramcontent.com/pod-product-compliance
Lightning Source LLC
Chambersburg PA
CBHW031122020426
42333CB00012B/187